My Grandmother's Witchy Medicine Cabinet

Disclaimer

The information and recipes contained in this book are based upon the research and the personal experiences of the author. It's for entertainment purposes only. It is not meant to replace any advice from a health care professional. This book is meant to compliment. The reader is encouraged to use good judgement when applying the information contained and to seek advice from a qualified professional if, and as needed. Professionals should be consulted as needed prior to undertaking any of the actions endorsed herein.

Every attempt has been made to provide accurate, up to date and reliable information. No warranties of any kind are expressed or implied. Readers acknowledge that the author is not engaging in the rendering of legal, financial, medical, or professional advice. By reading this, the reader agrees that under no circumstance the author is not responsible for any loss, direct or indirect, which is incurred by using this information contained within this book. Including but not limited to errors, omissions, or inaccuracies. This book is not intended as a replacement from what your health care provider has suggested. The author is not responsible for any adverse effects or consequences resulting from the use of any of the suggestions, preparations or procedures discussed in this book. All matters pertaining to your health should be supervised by a health care professional. I am not a doctor, or a medical professional nor do I play one on TV. This book is designed as an educational and entertainment tool only. Please always check with your health practitioner before taking any vitamins, supplements, diet change, or herbs, as they may have side-effects, especially when combined with medications, alcohol, or other vitamins or supplements.   Although every precaution has been taken by the author to verify the accuracy of the information contained herein, the author assumes no responsibility for any errors, or omissions. No liability is assumed for damages that may result from the information that is obtained within. The author declares that the research was conducted in the absence of any commercial or financial relationships that could be construed as a potential conflict of interest. This declaration is deemed fair and valid by both the American Bar association and the committee of publishers' association and is legally binding throughout the world.

By purchasing this book, you are consenting to its contents. It is important to note that the author of this book is not an expert on the topics discussed within, and any recommendations or suggestions made are for entertainment purposes only. It is recommended that professionals be consulted before taking any actions discussed in this book. This declaration has been deemed fair and valid by the American Bar Association and the Committee of Publishers' Association and is legally binding worldwide. The information contained in this book is considered truthful and accurate, and any use or misuse of the information is solely at the reader's discretion. The author cannot be held liable for any hardship or damages that may result from the reader's actions after reading this book.

A.L. Childers

All the data, research, footnotes, and references are cited in the back of the book, and it does back up all claims that have been discussed by the author. The internet is a valuable source of information, but unlike printed works, it cannot be relied upon for long-term reference. News articles may be removed from their websites, and data that you have cited may be erased, or the websites may have been terminated. This represents a challenge to authors who want to document the origin of their information.

Dear readers, it is important to take all necessary precautions before undertaking any DIY project. Always follow the instructions and be extra careful when creating your own homemade products. It is never a good idea to stretch yourself too thin. Remember that every fabric or material may react differently to suggested use. While this is a non-toxic and natural way to clean your home, it is always recommended to wear protective gloves and eyewear. Please note that although every effort has been made to provide you with the best possible information, neither the publisher nor the author is responsible for any accidents, injuries, or damage incurred because of tasks performed by readers. The author will not assume any responsibility for personal or property damage resulting from the formulas found in this book. It is important to keep in mind that this book is separate from professional services.

Authors note:

Please note that any reference or resemblance to any person or organization in this book, whether living or dead, existing, or defunct, is purely coincidental. I want to remind all readers that all rights are reserved and no part of this book or any associated ancillary materials may be reproduced or transmitted in any form by any means, electronic or mechanical, including photocopying, recording, duplicating, or by any informational storage or retrieval system, without express written permission from the author. It is important to respect the author's intellectual property and adhere to copyright laws.

A note of caution:

Prioritizing your own health and well-being is essential for a fulfilling life. I firmly believe that self-care and personal health empowerment are powerful tools, and that everyone should take the initiative to improve their own understanding. The more knowledge you have, the more control you have over your own health. However, it's important to remember that consulting with a trained medical professional is always necessary in cases of long-standing and undiagnosed symptoms. This book is not intended to replace professional medical judgment but can certainly serve as a valuable supplement to it. Stay informed and vigilant, but always remember to seek professional advice when needed. Please note that the information provided in this book is for educational and entertainment purposes only, and no warranty is given concerning the accuracy of this information. Be smart, be sensible, and prioritize your health by utilizing good common sense. Above all else, be kind and compassionate towards yourself, your body, and your mind.

An entity is different and specific to each individual or item to which it has attached itself. As to alternative forms of medicine or healing, the author of this book has yet to offer any promised outcomes. Some human issues are more profound than cleansing a new home or spiritual entity possession and removal. Therefore, you must understand that this isn't a quick fix for issues that may have gone on in your or someone else's life. Cleansing a new home or spiritual entity possession and removal is not designed as a replacement for traditional psychological and medical treatment or advice, and it is not intended to treat, diagnose, cure, or prevent any disease. There is a difference between entity removal, energy healing, deep-rooted physiological issues, and demonic possession. If you or someone you know seems to have signs of demonic activity, you should contact a priest for counsel and prayer. In addition, with the corporation and aid of a medical professional, they can help you discern if the symptoms have a more natural cause, physiological or physical. A priest can perform exorcisms if no such reasons can be clearly identified or if they seem to be occupied by a spirit. We don't need special authorization to perform deliverance prayers on a person, place, or object, but if it is an exorcism, you must have someone skilled and trained to perform it correctly.

All in all, a spiritual entity possession and entity attachment removal is not something you merely play around with. A demon will eat your lunch and pop that bag right before you.

As befitted in nature and a world that cannot be seen with human eyes, the author is protected by a binding spell of any malicious intent. Any dark or evil force may return to its source, shield my home, health, heart, and mind, as this includes all family, friends, objects, and animals of mine, as we remain free, always safe, and well indeed. You are bound to return to your source with flight; I banish thee with this holy light.

Dear Creator, please grant me your protection from those who attempt to justify evil actions as good and twist truth into lies to achieve their malicious intentions. I ask that you guard me and my loved ones against any forms of deceit and schemes against righteousness. May we be surrounded by the purest vibrations and a sphere of White Light that encompasses every corner, crack, and shelter of our dwellings. Please keep this sphere of White Light free from any negative or harmful energies, especially those of demonic origin. I also request that this sphere of White Light be expanded to cover the space that we always inhabit, ensuring our safety and well-being. Thank you for your guidance and protection.

Disclaimer:

In the enchanting world of "My Grandmother's Witchy Medicine Cabinet," we invite you on a journey through the realms of herbalism, connecting with ancient wisdom and the magic of nature. However, it is essential to recognize that the content provided in this exploration of holistic well-being is for informational and entertainment purposes only.

While we celebrate the rich heritage of herbal remedies and ancestral knowledge, it is imperative to consult with qualified healthcare professionals and experts before implementing any herbal practices or remedies. The information presented here should not be considered a substitute for professional medical advice, diagnosis, or treatment.

Furthermore, individual reactions to herbs and herbal remedies may vary, and it is crucial to exercise caution and discretion when incorporating them into your wellness routine. Any decision to use herbal remedies or engage in practices mentioned in this journey is made at your own discretion and risk.

We encourage you to seek guidance from healthcare providers and experts who can tailor advice and recommendations to your unique health needs. Your health and well-being are of utmost importance, and we wish for this exploration to serve as a source of inspiration and education on your path to holistic wellness.

By engaging with "My Grandmother's Witchy Medicine Cabinet," you acknowledge and accept this disclaimer, understanding that the content provided here is not intended to replace professional medical guidance.

Dear Readers,

I extend a warm and heartfelt welcome to you as you embark on this enchanting journey through the pages of "My Grandmother's Witchy Medicine Cabinet." As the author, I am both honored and excited to share with you the tales of my own childhood, filled with wonder and wisdom, as I discovered the magical world that thrived within my grandmother's forest, home and garden.

In the pages of this book, I invite you to step into a world where time seems to slow down, and the rhythm of nature sets the pace. My grandmother's garden, bathed in the soft glow of twilight, was more than just a collection of plants; it was a sanctuary where ancient knowledge converged with the vibrant energy of the natural world.

Growing up, I was fortunate to be surrounded by the soothing scents of herbs, the whispering leaves of ancient trees, and the gentle guidance of my grandmother's wisdom. Her medicine cabinet, filled with herbs, remedies, and the secrets of generations, was a treasure trove of healing magic.

Through the stories and experiences shared within these pages, I hope to transport you to that very garden, where you can feel the same sense of wonder and awe that I did as a child. Together, we will uncover the profound teachings of my grandmother and the ancient art of herbalism, a practice that she believed was intrinsically connected to our well-being.

As we journey through this book, remember that it is not just a collection of stories and knowledge but an opportunity for you to embrace the healing potential of the natural world. May you find inspiration, wisdom, and a renewed connection to the healing power of herbs and nature.

Thank you for joining me on this enchanting odyssey. May it be as transformative and enlightening for you as it has been for me.

With warmth and gratitude,

A. L. Childers

Introduction: Embracing the Healing Garden

In a world bustling with the clamor of modern life, there exists a timeless sanctuary—a place where ancient wisdom mingles with the vibrant pulse of nature, where the healing touch of the earth meets the yearning hearts of seekers, and where the legacy of generations past reaches out to embrace the present and future. This is the world of "My Grandmother's Witchy Medicine Cabinet," a journey through the art and magic of herbalism, guided by the wisdom passed down from one generation to the next.

As we embark on this enchanting odyssey, allow me to extend a warm invitation into a realm where herbal remedies are not just prescriptions, but pathways to holistic well-being. Picture a grandmother's garden bathed in the golden hues of a setting sun, where the gentle caress of the wind carries the whispers of plants that have witnessed centuries of healing and transformation. Here, among the fragrant herbs and vibrant blossoms, we will uncover the profound teachings of a grandmother who believed that the secrets of health and vitality are woven into the very fabric of the natural world.

Chapter 1: Seasons of Healing

Our journey begins with a deep dive into the rhythm of the seasons—a symphony orchestrated by the earth itself. In "Seasons of Healing," we will explore how nature's cycles influence our well-being and how the wisdom of herbs aligns with the ebb and flow of life. From the vibrant energies of spring to the restorative stillness of winter, we will discover the magic of herbalism as it harmonizes with the dance of the seasons.

Chapter 2: Roots of Wisdom

In "Roots of Wisdom," we delve into the heart of herbalism, where ancestral knowledge intertwines with the healing properties of plants. We'll unearth the stories of how our grandmothers and grandfathers nurtured the wisdom of herbal remedies, passing down the legacy that has become a treasure trove of natural healing. This chapter unveils the ancient roots of herbalism that continue to anchor our understanding of the power of the earth's offerings.

Chapter 3: The Art of Foraging

Venturing into the wilderness, we embark on a captivating exploration of "The Art of Foraging." In this chapter, we learn the age-old skill of gathering herbs directly from the wild. We'll roam through forests, meadows, and hidden corners of nature's bounty, discovering the secrets of identifying, harvesting, and respectfully foraging the plants that hold the keys to our well-being.

Chapter 4: From Garden to Table

A grandmother's garden is a treasure trove of healing, a living apothecary that beckons us to explore "From Garden to Table." In this chapter, we'll immerse ourselves in the enchanting world of cultivating our own herbs, creating a sanctuary where we can nurture our connection to the earth. Learn the art of growing, harvesting, and transforming these botanical wonders into potent remedies that not only heal the body but also touch the soul.

Chapter 5: The Alchemy of Herbal Blending

Prepare to unlock the secrets of "The Alchemy of Herbal Blending." Just as an artist blends colors to create a masterpiece, we, too, will explore the harmonious fusion of herbs to craft remedies with intention and creativity. The symphony of flavors, energies, and intentions will come together in a dance of synergy—a celebration of the artistry that is herbal blending.

Chapter 6: Herbs for the Heart and Soul

Herbalism is not just about physical health; it is a journey that encompasses the heart and soul. In "Herbs for the Heart and Soul," we will explore the emotional and spiritual dimensions of healing with herbs. From soothing herbal teas to potent elixirs, we will delve into remedies that nurture our inner landscape, bringing balance, joy, and serenity to our lives.

Chapter 7: Natural Remedies for Everyday Ailments

The journey of healing extends beyond the mystical to the practical. "Natural Remedies for Everyday Ailments" equips you with a toolkit of herbal remedies for common health challenges. From soothing sore throats to bolstering the immune system, we'll uncover the magic of herbs as they address the ailments that touch our daily lives.

Chapter 8: The Healing Garden: Cultivating Herbal Harmony

In this chapter, we will step into the heart of the healing garden, a sanctuary of intention and healing energies. "The Healing Garden: Cultivating Herbal Harmony" is an exploration of creating your own sacred space—a place where plants and people harmoniously coexist, and where the wisdom of the earth guides our journey toward holistic well-being.

Chapter 9: Herbal Wisdom for the Generations

The wisdom of herbalism is not ours to hoard but to share. "Herbal Wisdom for the Generations" invites you to become a steward of the herbal legacy, passing down the knowledge, stories, and traditions to future generations. Through journals, storytelling, mentorship, and teaching, we will ensure that the art of herbalism continues to thrive.

Chapter 10: The Healing Garden as a Legacy

As our journey concludes, we reflect on the legacy we leave behind. "The Healing Garden as a Legacy" explores the profound impact of cultivating a healing garden—a living entity that extends far beyond our own lifetimes. It is a reminder that herbalism is not just a practice but a way of life, a testament to our reverence for the earth and our commitment to holistic well-being.

So, dear reader, I invite you to journey with us through the pages of "My Grandmother's Witchy Medicine Cabinet." With each chapter, you will uncover the magic of herbalism—a world where the healing touch of nature meets the wisdom of generations, where the earth's offerings become our allies in the journey toward well-being, and where the legacy of herbal wisdom continues to flourish. Welcome to the enchanting world of herbalism—a journey of heart, soul, and the enduring magic of the healing garden.

Chapter 1: The Magical Medicine Cabinet

In the corner of my grandmother's cozy cottage, tucked away amidst the antique furniture and vintage trinkets, there stood a modest wooden cabinet. To most, it was just a piece of rustic furniture, but to me, it was nothing short of magical. My earliest memories are filled with the intrigue and wonder of that small, unassuming cupboard, which held the secrets of centuries-old wisdom and the healing power of nature.

As a child, I often found myself drawn to that enchanting medicine cabinet like a moth to a flame. It was a place of mystery and allure, filled with jars of dried herbs, amber-colored tinctures, and handwritten labels that seemed to whisper tales of healing and enchantment. But it was not the cabinet itself that held the magic; it was the knowledge and love that my grandmother poured into it.

The cabinet was a humble vessel, yet within its weathered wooden frame resided a treasure trove of herbal remedies and holistic cures that had been passed down through generations. It was a living testament to the ancient art of herbalism and the timeless wisdom of our ancestors. My grandmother, a wise woman in the truest sense of the word, was the guardian of this sacred knowledge.

Every summer, when the sun bathed our garden in golden warmth and the air was filled with the fragrance of blooming flowers, my grandmother would invite me to join her in the garden. She would beckon me with a smile that sparkled with both mischief and wisdom, and together, we would embark on a journey through the lush greenery that she had carefully nurtured for years.

"Come, child," she would say, her voice a soothing melody, "let me show you the magic of nature."

As we strolled among the rows of herbs and plants, she would introduce me to each one with reverence and affection, as if they were old friends. She would bend down to touch the leaves, releasing their aromatic oils into the air, and share stories of their healing properties. To me, these plants were no longer just botanical specimens; they were living beings with unique personalities and gifts.

My grandmother had a special connection with the earth and an intuitive understanding of the plants she tended. She knew when to sow the seeds, how to coax the herbs into flourishing, and when to harvest them for maximum potency. Her gardening practices were not just about growing plants; they were a dance of harmony between humans and nature, a partnership that had sustained our family for generations.

One sunny afternoon, as we stood amidst the towering sunflowers and fragrant lavender, my grandmother turned to me and said, "Child, these plants are not merely for decoration. They are our allies in health and healing. They are the key to unlocking the body's innate ability to restore balance and vitality."

With those words, she opened the door to a world of natural remedies and holistic health that would shape my life in profound ways. She taught me the art of harvesting and drying herbs, showing me how to carefully pluck leaves, flowers, and roots at the peak of their potency. In her gentle, patient way, she explained the importance of gratitude and intention in every step of the process.

"Each herb has a purpose, a story, and a spirit," she would say. "When we harvest with respect and gratitude, we honor the plant's sacrifice and harness its healing energy."

Back in the cottage, the magic continued. The modest medicine cabinet became our alchemical laboratory, where we transformed dried herbs into potent potions and tinctures. My grandmother's hands moved with grace and precision as she measured, mixed, and infused herbs with love and intention. Her recipes were a blend of ancient wisdom and intuition, passed down through generations of healers.

One of my fondest memories is watching her create a soothing lavender salve. She carefully melted beeswax and mixed it with lavender-infused oil, creating a fragrant balm that would soothe skin irritations and calm the senses. As she poured the warm liquid into small glass jars, she looked at me with eyes that held a deep knowing.

"This salve," she explained, "is not just for physical healing. It carries the essence of the lavender plant, which brings peace and tranquility to the soul. Remember, healing is not only about the body; it's about nurturing the spirit as well."

My grandmother's teachings extended beyond the physical realm. She believed in the profound connection between mind, body, and spirit—a holistic approach to health that transcended conventional medicine. She introduced me to meditation, mindfulness, and the power of positive affirmations. Together, we would sit in the garden, surrounded by the symphony of nature's sounds, and she would guide me in a journey of inner exploration.

"Quiet your mind, dear one," she would say. "Listen to the wisdom that resides within you. Your body knows how to heal itself if you give it the space and stillness to do so."

Under her guidance, I learned to embrace the mind-body connection and the importance of emotional well-being in the healing process. It was a lesson that would serve me well throughout my life, as I discovered the profound impact of stress, emotions, and beliefs on my health.

My grandmother's holistic approach to health was not limited to the physical and emotional aspects; it also encompassed the spiritual dimension. She believed that we were all connected to a larger tapestry of life, and that our well-being was intimately linked to the natural world. She would often speak of the Earth as a generous mother who provided us with everything we needed for healing and sustenance.

"Nature is our greatest healer," she would say, her eyes gazing at the vast expanse of the garden. "The plants, the trees, the rivers—they hold the secrets to our vitality and harmony. We are but one thread in the intricate web of life."

As I listened to her words, I couldn't help but feel a deep sense of awe and gratitude for the world around me. I began to see the interconnectedness of all living beings and the importance of respecting and preserving the delicate balance of nature.

The lessons my grandmother imparted to me extended far beyond the garden and the medicine cabinet. She shared her wisdom not only through words but also through the tangible results of her herbal remedies. Over the years, I witnessed countless instances of healing and transformation in our family and community.

From soothing chamomile tea that eased the restlessness of sleepless nights to potent ginger tinctures that provided relief from digestive discomfort, my grandmother's herbal remedies touched the lives of many. Friends and neighbors would often seek her guidance, and she would graciously share her knowledge and remedies, never asking for anything in return.

One winter, when a severe flu outbreak swept through our town, my grandmother's kitchen became a refuge for the sick and weary. She brewed herbal teas, prepared nourishing soups, and offered comforting words of encouragement. Her healing touch and the power of her remedies brought solace to those in need.

It was during these moments of witnessing the profound impact of her work that I realized the true magic of my grandmother's medicine cabinet. It wasn't just a collection of herbs and potions; it was a symbol of love, compassion, and the timeless wisdom of generations past. It was a testament to the healing potential that resides within each of us and the bountiful gifts that nature provides.

As I grew older, my bond with my grandmother deepened, and the lessons she imparted became an integral part of my life.

1. **Springtime Renewal Herbal Tea**

Ingredients:

1 tablespoon fresh nettle leaves

1 tablespoon fresh dandelion leaves

1 tablespoon fresh peppermint leaves

Honey to taste

Boiling water

Instructions:

In a teapot, combine the nettle, dandelion, and peppermint leaves.

Pour boiling water over the herbs and let steep for 5-7 minutes.

Sweeten with honey to your liking.

Sip slowly, feeling the rejuvenating energy of spring flow through you. Remember that just as the earth awakens, so can you.

2. **Summer Solstice Sunshine Soup**

Ingredients:

2 cups sunflower petals

1 cup fresh basil leaves

2 ripe tomatoes, chopped

1 small red onion, finely diced

4 cups vegetable broth

Salt and pepper to taste

Instructions:

In a pot, bring the vegetable broth to a simmer.

Add sunflower petals, basil leaves, chopped tomatoes, and diced red onion.

Simmer for 15-20 minutes until the flavors meld.

Season with salt and pepper to taste.

Savor this vibrant soup as it warms your heart, celebrating the abundance of summer.

3. **Autumn Harvest Stew**

Ingredients:

2 cups butternut squash, cubed

1 cup sliced mushrooms

1 cup kale leaves, torn

1 medium onion, chopped

4 cups vegetable broth

1 teaspoon dried sage

Salt and pepper to taste

Instructions:

In a large pot, combine all the ingredients.

Bring to a gentle boil, then reduce heat to a simmer.

Let the stew simmer for 25-30 minutes until the squash is tender.

Season with sage, salt, and pepper.

As you enjoy this nourishing stew, remember that change is natural, and like the falling leaves, it's a part of life's cycle.

4. **Winter's Embrace Healing Tea**

Ingredients:

1 tablespoon dried chamomile flowers

1 tablespoon dried lavender buds

1 teaspoon dried rosemary

1 teaspoon honey

Boiling water

Instructions:

Combine chamomile, lavender, and rosemary in a teapot.

Pour boiling water over the herbs and steep for 5-7 minutes.

Add honey to taste.

Sip slowly, allowing the warmth of this tea to envelop you. Remember that rest and introspection are vital during the winter months.

5. **Spring Blossom Salad**

Ingredients:

2 cups fresh mixed spring greens

1/2 cup edible flower petals (violets, pansies, nasturtiums)

1/4 cup fresh chive blossoms

Lemon vinaigrette (lemon juice, olive oil, honey)

Instructions:

Toss the spring greens, edible flower petals, and chive blossoms in a bowl.

Drizzle with lemon vinaigrette.

Enjoy this vibrant salad as a reminder of the beauty that emerges with the changing seasons.

6. **Summer Berry Elixir**

Ingredients:

1 cup fresh mixed berries (strawberries, blueberries, raspberries)

1 tablespoon fresh lemon balm leaves

1 teaspoon raw honey

2 cups cold water

Instructions:

In a blender, combine berries, lemon balm leaves, honey, and cold water.

Blend until smooth.

Strain the mixture to remove seeds.

Sip on this refreshing elixir and feel the vitality of summer flowing through you.

7. **Autumn Comforting Porridge**

Ingredients:

1 cup rolled oats

2 cups goats milk (or any preferred milk)

1/2 cup chopped apples

1/4 cup chopped walnuts

1 teaspoon cinnamon

1 tablespoon maple syrup

Instructions:

In a saucepan, combine oats and almond milk. Bring to a simmer.

Add chopped apples, walnuts, and cinnamon.

Cook until the porridge thickens and the apples soften.

Sweeten with maple syrup.

Savor this warm and nourishing porridge, knowing that like the trees shedding their leaves, it's okay to let go of what no longer serves you.

8. **Winter Solstice Root Soup**

Ingredients:

2 cups diced root vegetables (carrots, parsnips, turnips)

1 cup leeks, sliced

4 cups vegetable broth

1 teaspoon thyme

Salt and pepper to taste

Instructions:

In a pot, combine root vegetables, leeks, and vegetable broth.

Bring to a boil, then reduce heat and simmer for 20-25 minutes until the vegetables are tender.

Season with thyme, salt, and pepper.

As you enjoy this hearty soup, find comfort in the quiet strength of winter's embrace.

9. **Springtime Herbal Infusion**

Ingredients:

A handful of fresh lemon balm leaves

A handful of fresh calendula petals

Boiling water

Instructions:

Place lemon balm leaves and calendula petals in a teapot.

Pour boiling water over them and steep for 10-15 minutes.

Sip this soothing infusion as a reminder that even after the darkest of winters, the light of spring always returns.

In my grandmother's tradition, words of encouragement are as important as her healing recipes. Remember that life, like the seasons, goes through cycles. During moments of change or challenge, find strength in her wisdom:

"Like the earth, you too have seasons. Embrace the growth of spring, the warmth of summer, the reflection of autumn, and the rest of winter. Each phase has its purpose and beauty. Trust in the cycles of life, and you will find your own healing."

"May the herbs from our garden and the wisdom of generations past guide you on your journey. Just as the seasons change, so can you transform and heal."

"Know that in every challenge, there is an opportunity for growth. Like the herbs in our garden, you have the power to bloom and thrive, no matter the season."

As you explore the "Seasons of Healing," may these recipes and words of encouragement guide you on your own journey of well-being and self-discovery, just as your grandmother's wisdom has done for generations.

Chapter 2: Grandma's Green Thumb: Growing Natural Remedies

In the heart of our family's ancestral home, nestled within the embrace of rolling hills and the gentle curve of a meandering river, lay a garden that was unlike any other. It was a garden that breathed with life, whispered with secrets, and sang with the healing melodies of nature. This sacred space, carefully tended by my grandmother, was a living testament to her profound connection with the earth and her mastery of the art of cultivating herbs and plants for healing.

As a child, I often marveled at the way my grandmother's green thumb seemed to possess an almost magical touch. She could coax life from the soil with a mere whisper, nurturing plants with a tenderness that only a true steward of the land could understand. To me, this garden was a realm of enchantment, where the ordinary became extraordinary, and the mundane was transformed into something sacred.

"Come, my dear," my grandmother would say, her eyes twinkling with mischief and anticipation. "Let us step into the garden, where magic and medicine await."

Our journeys into the garden were a cherished ritual—a dance of harmony between humans and nature, a partnership that had sustained our family for generations. The garden, you see, was not just a place to grow pretty flowers and aromatic herbs; it was a living pharmacy, a sanctuary of healing, and a classroom of wisdom.

With each step we took on the cobblestone path that wound through the garden, my grandmother introduced me to the various inhabitants of this green kingdom. Each plant had its own story, its own personality, and its own gift to offer. She taught me to approach them with respect and reverence, as if they were elders with centuries of wisdom to impart.

The first stop on our botanical journey was the towering sunflowers that stood sentinel at the garden's entrance. Their bright, golden faces turned toward the sun, soaking in its warmth and radiance. My grandmother explained that the sunflower represented vitality and strength, a symbol of the sun's life-giving energy.

"Sunflowers," she said, "remind us of the importance of embracing the light within ourselves. Just as they follow the sun's path across the sky, we too must seek the light of knowledge and self-discovery."

As we continued our exploration, we encountered the fragrant lavender bushes, their purple blooms dancing in the breeze. My grandmother's fingers brushed against the soft, aromatic leaves, releasing a symphony of lavender's soothing scent.

"Lavender," she told me, "Is a gentle healer of both body and spirit. Its essence calms the mind, eases stress, and invites peaceful sleep. It is a reminder that even in the midst of chaos, there is a sanctuary of tranquility within us."

We ventured deeper into the garden, where rows of rosemary bushes thrived. Their woody stems and needle-like leaves exuded a fragrant and invigorating aroma. My grandmother shared stories of rosemary's significance in ancient traditions, where it symbolized remembrance and fidelity.

"Rosemary," she explained, "is not only a culinary delight but also a guardian of memory and clarity. Its presence in our garden reminds us to honor our past, embrace our heritage, and stay true to our roots."

The garden was a vibrant tapestry of colors, scents, and textures. Each plant had its purpose, and my grandmother knew them intimately. She could discern the subtlest changes in the leaves, the slightest shift in the soil's moisture, and the whispers of the wind as it rustled through the leaves. Her connection with the garden was a silent conversation—a communion of energy and intention.

As the seasons cycled through their graceful dance, the garden transformed in response to the rhythms of nature. Spring brought forth a riot of blossoms—vivid tulips, delicate violets, and cheerful daffodils. Summer's warmth awakened the aromatic herbs, while autumn painted the landscape with a palette of fiery reds and oranges. Even in the depths of winter, when snow blanketed the earth, the garden slumbered, gathering its strength for the rebirth of spring.

My grandmother's approach to gardening was a blend of ancient wisdom and intuitive knowledge. She understood the importance of planting with intention, aligning the garden's energy with the cycles of the moon, and respecting the natural order of growth and decay. Her hands moved with a grace born of years of practice, and she knew when to prune, when to water, and when to let the garden breathe.

"Every action we take in the garden," she would say, "is a dance of energy and intention. We are co-creators with nature, and our role is to listen, observe, and nurture."

One of the most profound lessons my grandmother imparted to me was the art of harvesting herbs and plants. It was a skill that required not only knowledge but also a deep connection with the plants themselves. She emphasized the importance of harvesting at the peak of potency, when the plant's energy and vitality were at their zenith.

"Imagine," she would say, "that you are offering gratitude to the plant for its gift of healing. Approach it with respect, speak to it in whispers, and ask for its permission to harvest."

With her guidance, I learned to carefully pluck leaves, flowers, and roots, taking only what was needed and leaving the rest to thrive. We would gather our harvest in woven baskets, the vibrant colors and fragrant scents mingling to create a sensory symphony.

Back in the cottage, the magic of the garden continued. The humble medicine cabinet transformed into an alchemical laboratory where we transformed our bounty of herbs into potent remedies. My grandmother's hands moved with a grace that was both skillful and reverent as she measured, mixed, and infused herbs with love and intention.

One summer's day, as the golden rays of the sun streamed through the window, my grandmother taught me to create a soothing chamomile tea. She carefully measured dried chamomile flowers and placed them in a porcelain teapot, her movements deliberate and precise.

"Chamomile," she explained, "is a gentle healer of the digestive system and a comforter of restless souls. It brings the warmth of the sun into our bodies and soothes the storm within."

As the tea steeped, filling the room with its calming fragrance, my grandmother poured it into delicate china cups. We sat together, sipping the golden elixir, and she shared stories of chamomile's ancient use as a remedy for sleeplessness and anxiety.

"This tea," she said, "is not just a beverage; it is a balm for the spirit. It reminds us to find solace in simplicity and to embrace the healing power of nature's gifts."

The garden, you see, was not just a place of physical nourishment; it was a wellspring of wisdom and a source of spiritual sustenance. In its lush embrace, I learned that the act of growing herbs and plants was more than a mere agricultural endeavor—it was a sacred practice, a communion with the earth, and a reminder of our interconnectedness with all of creation.

As the years passed, my bond with my grandmother deepened, and the lessons she imparted became an integral part of my life. I came to understand that the garden was not only a place of healing but also a sanctuary of memories, a testament to the enduring legacy of our ancestors, and a living testament to the timeless wisdom of herbalism.

In the garden, my grandmother had sown the seeds of knowledge, and in my heart, they had taken root. The lessons of cultivation, intention, and reverence for the earth would shape my path in profound ways, leading me to embrace the healing power of nature and the wisdom of generations past.

1. Grandma's Comforting Chamomile Tea

Ingredients:

1 tablespoon dried chamomile flowers

1 cup boiling water

Honey (optional)

Instructions:

Place the dried chamomile flowers in a teapot.

Pour boiling water over the flowers and let steep for 5-7 minutes.

Add honey to taste if desired.

Sip slowly, and let the calming warmth of chamomile soothe your soul.

Words of Wisdom: "Child, when life feels stormy, remember that just as chamomile blooms despite adversity, you too can find peace in the midst of chaos."

2. **Elderberry Elixir for Immunity**

Ingredients:

1/2 cup dried elderberries

2 cups water

1 cup honey

1 lemon, sliced

Instructions:

In a saucepan, combine elderberries and water. Bring to a boil.

Reduce heat and simmer for 30 minutes.

Strain the liquid into a jar, add honey, and stir until well combined.

Add lemon slices for an extra boost.

Take a spoonful when you need to strengthen your immunity.

Words of Wisdom: "Like the elderberry tree, which stands strong through the seasons, remember to nurture your health and inner strength."

3. Healing Calendula Salve

Ingredients:

1/2 cup dried calendula petals

1 cup olive oil

Beeswax (for consistency)

Instructions:

Place dried calendula petals in a glass jar.

Cover with olive oil, ensuring the petals are fully submerged.

Seal the jar and let it sit in a sunny spot for 2-4 weeks.

Strain the infused oil and mix with melted beeswax to create a salve.

Apply to minor cuts, burns, or dry skin for healing.

Words of Wisdom: "Just as calendula blooms even in harsh conditions, you possess the inner strength to heal and nurture those around you."

4. Lavender Dream Pillow

Ingredients:

Dried lavender flowers

A small muslin bag or pillowcase

Instructions:

Fill a small muslin bag or pillowcase with dried lavender flowers.

Place it under your pillow.

Inhale the soothing scent as you drift into peaceful slumber.

Words of Wisdom: "Child, let the sweet scent of lavender carry away your worries and invite dreams of hope and happiness."

5. Sage and Rosemary Smudge Bundle

Ingredients:

Dried sage leaves

Dried rosemary sprigs

String or twine

Instructions:

Bundle dried sage leaves and rosemary sprigs together, tying them with string.

Light the bundle and allow it to smolder, releasing purifying smoke.

Use the smoke to cleanse your space and spirit.

Words of Wisdom: "As sage and rosemary purify the air, let go of negativity and embrace the cleansing power of love and positivity."

6. **Juniper Berry Bath Soak**

Ingredients:

Handful of dried juniper berries

Epsom salt

Lavender essential oil (optional)

Instructions:

Add dried juniper berries and Epsom salt to a warm bath.

Optional: Add a few drops of lavender essential oil.

Soak and allow the healing properties of juniper to wash over you.

Words of Wisdom: "Just as the juniper tree thrives in rocky soil, you can overcome challenges and grow stronger through life's trials."

7. Rose Petal Syrup

Ingredients:

1 cup fresh rose petals (unsprayed)

1 cup water

1 cup sugar

Instructions:

In a saucepan, combine rose petals, water, and sugar.

Simmer for 15-20 minutes until the petals lose their color.

Strain the syrup into a glass jar.

Use as a sweet topping for desserts or mix with water for a floral drink.

Words of Wisdom: "Child, just as roses bloom with grace and fragrance, let your actions and words carry beauty and kindness into the world."

8. Yarrow Wound Poultice

Ingredients:

Fresh yarrow leaves and flowers

Clean cloth

Instructions:

Crush fresh yarrow leaves and flowers.

Place them on a clean cloth.

Apply the poultice to minor cuts or wounds to aid in healing and prevent infection.

Words of Wisdom: "Like yarrow's ability to staunch bleeding, remember that you have the strength to mend your own wounds."

9. Sage and Thyme Herbal Hair Rinse

Ingredients:

Handful of dried sage leaves

Handful of dried thyme leaves

2 cups boiling water

Instructions:

Combine dried sage and thyme in a large bowl.

Pour boiling water over the herbs and let steep until it cools.

Strain and use as a final rinse after shampooing your hair.

Words of Wisdom: "Child, just as herbs nourish your hair, take care of yourself and your natural beauty will shine."

10. Words of Wisdom

As my grandmother would gently remind me:

"Dear one, the roots of our wisdom run deep, just like the earth's foundation. Embrace the knowledge passed down through generations, for it holds the key to healing, strength, and connection with the natural world. Keep these traditions alive, and may they guide you on your journey with love and resilience."

Chapter 3: Learning from the Earth: Herbal Wisdom

The sun hung low on the horizon, casting a warm, golden glow across the garden. It was a tranquil afternoon, and my grandmother and I sat on a weathered wooden bench, surrounded by the lush greenery that was her pride and joy. The garden had become a place of solace and learning, a living testament to the wisdom of generations and the enduring magic of nature.

As I leaned in closer to my grandmother, I couldn't help but feel a sense of anticipation. Her eyes sparkled with the wisdom of ages, and her gentle smile held the promise of ancient secrets about to be unveiled.

"Today," she began, her voice a melodious whisper, "we shall embark on a journey into the heart of herbal wisdom—the profound knowledge that has been passed down through generations of healers, wise women, and herbalists."

With those words, she opened a gateway to a world that was as old as humanity itself. It was a world where plants were not just green entities rooted in the earth, but living beings with their own stories, personalities, and healing gifts.

"Herbal wisdom," my grandmother continued, "is the art of understanding and harnessing the healing power of plants. It is a dance of intuition, observation, and reverence for the natural world."

As I sat beside her, I felt the weight of centuries of tradition and the depth of ancestral knowledge that she carried. She was not just a gardener; she was a guardian of ancient wisdom—a torchbearer of the herbal traditions that had sustained our family for generations.

"Let us begin," she said, her eyes fixed on a cluster of vibrant calendula blossoms that swayed in the breeze. "Calendula, also known as 'marigold,' is a plant of great significance in herbal medicine. Its bright, sunny petals carry the energy of healing and rejuvenation."

My grandmother plucked a handful of calendula flowers and held them up to the sunlight. Their vivid orange hue seemed to capture the very essence of vitality.

"Calendula," she explained, "is a versatile herb with a wide range of healing properties. Its vibrant color symbolizes its ability to bring warmth and light to the body and soul. It is a gentle but powerful ally in our herbal repertoire."

As she spoke, my grandmother's hands moved with a grace born of years of practice. She carefully harvested the calendula blossoms, ensuring that each one was chosen with intention and gratitude. It was a lesson in mindfulness—a reminder that every action in the world of herbalism should be imbued with reverence for nature's gifts.

We returned to the cottage, where the familiar medicine cabinet awaited us. My grandmother placed the freshly harvested calendula blossoms on a clean wooden surface and began the process of drying them. She spread them out in a single layer, ensuring that they had ample space to breathe and release their moisture.

"Drying herbs," she said, "is a crucial step in preserving their potency. It allows us to capture the essence of the plant and store it for future use."

The gentle hum of a ceiling fan wafted through the room, aiding in the drying process. My grandmother explained that air circulation was essential to prevent mold and ensure the herbs' quality.

"Drying herbs," she continued, "is akin to the art of patience. We must give the plants the time they need to release their energy and transform into healing allies."

As we waited for the calendula blossoms to dry, my grandmother shared stories of the generations of herbalists who had come before us. She spoke of wise women who were revered in their communities for their knowledge of plant medicine, of shamans who communed with the spirits of the forest, and of healers who understood the intricate dance between the natural world and human health.

"Herbalism," she said, "is a thread that weaves through the tapestry of human history. It is a tradition that transcends cultures and continents, a universal language spoken by those who seek healing and harmony."

With the calendula blossoms now thoroughly dried, my grandmother carefully placed them in a glass jar. She sealed the jar with a cork stopper and labeled it with elegant handwriting, marking the date of harvest and the name of the herb.

"Labeling," she emphasized, "is a practice of respect for the plant and a way to honor its contribution to our well-being. It ensures that we can identify and appreciate the herbs we work with."

I watched in awe as my grandmother's hands moved with a sense of purpose and reverence. The simple act of preserving the calendula blossoms felt like a sacred ritual—an acknowledgment of the deep connection between humanity and the natural world.

With the calendula jar safely stored in the medicine cabinet, my grandmother turned her attention to a collection of dried herbs and roots that lined one of the cabinet's shelves.

"Each herb," she said, "has its own unique energy and healing properties. To become a true herbalist, one must learn to listen to the whispers of the plants, to understand their language, and to use their gifts wisely."

She selected a small bundle of dried sage leaves and crumbled them into a ceramic bowl. The earthy aroma filled the room, and I closed my eyes, inhaling deeply, allowing the scent to envelop me.

"Sage," my grandmother explained, "is a plant of purification and clarity. Its cleansing properties are not only physical but also spiritual. It has been used for centuries to clear negative energy and bring wisdom to those who seek it."

She placed the crumbled sage leaves into a small, heatproof dish and lit them with a match. The leaves smoldered, releasing a fragrant smoke that wafted upward, filling the room with a sense of sacredness.

"Smudging," she said, "is a practice of clearing and consecrating a space or an individual. The smoke of sage carries our intentions and prayers, allowing us to create a sacred atmosphere."

My grandmother walked around the room, holding the smoldering sage dish with a feather. The feather acted as a gentle fan, directing the smoke into every corner and crevice. As she moved with grace and purpose, it was as though she was weaving a protective cocoon of energy around us.

"Smudging," she continued, "is a way of acknowledging the spiritual dimension of healing. It is a reminder that true health encompasses not only the physical body but also the soul."

As I watched her perform the smudging ritual, I felt a profound sense of connection to something greater than myself. It was as though the room itself had come alive, resonating with the energy of the herbs and the intention of the ceremony.

My grandmother concluded the smudging ritual and returned the sage dish to its place in the medicine cabinet. She then turned her attention to a small bundle of dried lavender flowers, which she carefully tied together with a piece of twine.

"Lavender," she said, "is a plant of peace and serenity. Its soothing aroma calms the mind and invites relaxation. It is a gentle but potent ally in our quest for emotional well-being."

She instructed me to hang the bundle of lavender by a window, where it would catch the soft, diffused light of the setting sun. The lavender would gradually release its fragrance, infusing the room with a sense of tranquility.

"Herbs," my grandmother explained, "have a language of their own. They speak to us through their scents, their colors, and their energies. Learning to understand and interpret that language is the essence of herbal wisdom."

As we sat in the room filled with the delicate scent of lavender, my grandmother shared stories of her own journey into the world of herbalism. She spoke of her mentors—wise women and herbalists who had guided her path and shared their knowledge.

"I was fortunate," she said, her eyes reflecting a deep sense of gratitude, "to have been mentored by women who understood the sacredness of herbal medicine. They taught me not only the practical aspects of working with herbs but also the importance of intuition and connection."

Her herbal mentors had passed down not only knowledge but also a sense of responsibility—a duty to preserve and carry forward the traditions of healing. They had instilled in her a deep reverence for the natural world and a commitment to sharing her wisdom with others.

"I, in turn," she said, "have the honor of passing this knowledge on to you, my dear. It is a legacy that spans generations—a torch that is entrusted to those who will carry it forward."

As I listened to my grandmother's words, I realized the weight of the knowledge that had been placed in my hands. It was a responsibility that I embraced with humility and awe—a commitment to honor the wisdom of the plants, the traditions of herbalism, and the bond that connected us to the earth.

In the days and weeks that followed, my grandmother continued to teach me the intricacies of herbalism—the art of formulation, the understanding of energetics, and the practice of creating remedies that addressed both the physical and spiritual aspects of healing. Each lesson was a step deeper into the world of herbal wisdom, a world that held the keys to health, harmony, and the enduring magic of nature.

As I look back on those precious moments with my grandmother, I realize that the essence of herbal wisdom is not merely about the accumulation of facts and information; it is about a profound connection with the natural world, a deep respect for the plants that sustain us, and a commitment to the ancient traditions that have stood the test of time.

In the pages of my grandmother's teachings, I discovered a treasure trove of knowledge that would shape my path and guide my journey into the world of herbalism. It was a journey that transcended the boundaries of time and space, weaving together the wisdom of generations past and the promise of a future filled with healing, harmony, and reverence for the earth.

As we sat in the garden on that tranquil afternoon, the sun dipping below the horizon, I couldn't help but feel a profound sense of gratitude—for the lessons imparted, for the wisdom shared, and for the enduring magic of herbalism that had become an inseparable part of my life. The garden, the medicine cabinet, and the herbal wisdom they held were not just elements of my past; they were the guiding stars of my future, illuminating the path to a deeper understanding of the healing power of nature and the interconnectedness of all living beings.

1. Wild Nettle and Dandelion Soup

Ingredients:

2 cups fresh nettle leaves (wear gloves when handling)

1 cup fresh dandelion greens

1 small onion, chopped

2 cloves garlic, minced

4 cups vegetable broth

Salt and pepper to taste

Instructions:

Carefully gather nettle leaves and dandelion greens.

In a pot, sauté onion and garlic until fragrant.

Add nettle leaves, dandelion greens, and vegetable broth.

Simmer for 15-20 minutes until greens are tender.

Season with salt and pepper.

Enjoy the nourishing flavors of the wild.

Words of Wisdom: "Child, just as we learn to respect the wild plants, remember to respect the world around you. Nature has much to teach us if we listen."

2. Elderflower Cordial

Ingredients:

20 elderflower heads

4 cups water

4 cups sugar

2 lemons, thinly sliced

2 tablespoons citric acid

Instructions:

Gather elderflower heads from the wild.

In a large bowl, combine water and sugar, stirring until dissolved.

Add elderflowers, lemon slices, and citric acid.

Cover and let sit for 2-3 days.

Strain and bottle the fragrant cordial.

Serve with sparkling water for a refreshing drink.

Words of Wisdom: "Much like the elderflowers in the wild, remember to savor the simple pleasures in life. They are the sweetest."

3. **Wild Rose Petal Elixir**

Ingredients:

Fresh wild rose petals (unsprayed)

Honey

Brandy (optional)

Instructions:

Collect fragrant wild rose petals.

Place them in a glass jar and cover with honey.

Optional: Add a splash of brandy for preservation.

Let the petals infuse for several weeks.

Use a few drops as a mood-lifting elixir.

Words of Wisdom: "Child, just as the wild roses share their beauty freely, let your love and kindness bloom without reservation."

4. **Forest Mushroom Risotto**

Ingredients:

2 cups foraged wild mushrooms (chanterelles, porcini, morels)

1 1/2 cups Arborio rice

1/2 cup white wine

4 cups vegetable broth

1 onion, chopped

2 cloves garlic, minced

Fresh thyme

Parmesan cheese (optional)

Olive oil

Salt and pepper to taste

Instructions:

Clean and slice the wild mushrooms.

Sauté onions and garlic in olive oil.

Add mushrooms and cook until tender.

Stir in Arborio rice and cook for a few minutes.

Pour in white wine and allow it to absorb.

Gradually add vegetable broth, stirring until the rice is creamy.

Season with thyme, salt, and pepper.

Optional: Serve with Parmesan cheese.

Words of Wisdom: "Like the mushrooms hidden in the forest, life's treasures are often discovered when you venture beyond your comfort zone."

The recipe for Forest Mushroom Risotto includes instructions on foraging wild mushrooms, which can be an enjoyable and rewarding experience. However, it is crucial to exercise extreme caution when foraging for wild mushrooms, as not all mushrooms are safe for consumption. Some wild mushrooms can be toxic and pose serious health risks, including life-threatening conditions.

Foraging Safety Tips:

Expertise: Ensure that you have sufficient knowledge and experience in identifying edible mushrooms accurately. If you are uncertain about the identification of any mushroom species, do not consume it.

Consult an Expert: It is highly recommended to consult with a mycologist or an experienced forager who can guide you in identifying safe and edible wild mushrooms.

Local Regulations: Be aware of any local regulations regarding foraging for wild mushrooms. Some areas may have restrictions or require permits.

Avoid Risky Varieties: Do not attempt to forage for mushrooms that are known to be toxic, or closely resemble toxic species.

Double-Check: Always double-check the identification of mushrooms using reputable field guides or online resources.

Children and Pets: Keep children and pets away from foraged mushrooms, as they may be more susceptible to mushroom poisoning.

Allergies and Sensitivities: Be mindful of any allergies or sensitivities you may have to mushrooms.

Cook Thoroughly: Ensure that all wild mushrooms are cooked thoroughly before consumption, as some toxins may be neutralized by cooking.

Liability:

The author of this recipe and the platform providing this information are not responsible for any harm, illness, or adverse effects that may result from foraging, preparing, or consuming wild mushrooms. Individuals choosing to forage for wild mushrooms do so at their own risk and should exercise the utmost caution, seek expert guidance, and use their best judgment.

Words of Wisdom:

"Like the mushrooms hidden in the forest, life's treasures are often discovered when you venture beyond your comfort zone. Remember, in all aspects of life, safety, wisdom, and care should guide your journey."

5. **Chickweed Healing Salve**

Ingredients:

Fresh chickweed leaves and flowers

Olive oil

Beeswax

Instructions:

Gather fresh chickweed.

Place chickweed in a glass jar and cover with olive oil.

Let it sit in the sun for 2-4 weeks.

Strain the infused oil and mix with melted beeswax to create a salve.

Apply to minor skin irritations and enjoy its soothing properties.

Words of Wisdom: "Child, just as chickweed soothes the skin, remember that kindness and compassion soothe the soul."

6. Forest Berry Jam

Ingredients:

Foraged wild berries (blackberries, raspberries, strawberries)

Sugar

Lemon juice

Instructions:

Collect wild berries.

Place them in a saucepan with an equal amount of sugar.

Add a splash of lemon juice.

Cook until the mixture thickens.

Allow the jam to cool and store in jars.

Words of Wisdom: "Much like the wild berries, the sweetest moments in life are often found when you least expect them."

7. **Wild Mint and Lemon Balm Tea**

Ingredients:

Fresh wild mint leaves

Fresh lemon balm leaves

Boiling water

Instructions:

Gather wild mint and lemon balm leaves from your foraging adventure.

Place the leaves in a teapot.

Pour boiling water over them and steep for 5-7 minutes.

Sip slowly, savoring the refreshing flavors of the wild.

Words of Wisdom: "Child, like the wild mint and lemon balm, let your spirit remain fresh and invigorated even in the face of challenges."

8. **Pine Needle Syrup**

Ingredients:

Fresh pine needles (young, tender shoots)

Sugar

Water

Instructions:

Collect fresh pine needles.

Place them in a saucepan with sugar and water.

Simmer until the liquid thickens to a syrupy consistency.

Strain and store the syrup.

Use as a natural remedy for coughs and sore throats.

Words of Wisdom: "Just as the pine trees stand tall and unwavering, may you find strength in your own resilience."

9. Elderberry and Hawthorn Berry Tonic

Ingredients:

Fresh elderberries

Fresh hawthorn berries

Honey (optional)

Instructions:

Gather fresh elderberries and hawthorn berries.

Mash the berries and strain the juice.

Add honey to taste, if desired.

Sip on this tonic to boost your heart health and immunity.

Words of Wisdom: "Child, like the elderberries and hawthorn berries, may your heart remain healthy and your spirit resilient."

10. **Words of Wisdom**

As my grandmother would lovingly remind me:

"Dear one, foraging in the wild teaches us the importance of patience, respect, and connection with the earth. Remember that life, like nature, has a delicate balance. Embrace the treasures you discover, for they hold the wisdom of generations past and the promise of a vibrant future."

With every step you take in "The Art of Foraging," may you not only discover the bounty of nature but also the richness of your own journey. Be mindful, be curious, and let the whispers of the wild guide you on your path to well-being and wisdom.

Smudging is a ceremonial practice that involves burning herbs, typically sage or a combination of herbs, to purify and cleanse the energy of a space, object, or person. Here's how to perform a basic smudging ritual:

Materials Needed:

A bundle of dried white sage or a smudging blend that includes lavender and sage.

A heat-resistant bowl or shell to catch ashes.

A feather, fan, or your hand to waft the smoke.

A lighter or matches.

Steps:

Prepare Your Space: Ensure you are in a calm and quiet environment where you won't be disturbed. Open windows or doors to allow any negative energy to leave the space.

Light the Sage: Hold one end of the sage bundle over the bowl or shell and use a lighter or matches to ignite the other end. Allow it to burn for a few seconds, then gently blow out the flame so that the sage smolders and produces smoke.

Set Your Intention: Before you start smudging, take a moment to set your intention. This could be a specific purpose, such as clearing negativity, inviting positive energy, or blessing a space.

Begin Smudging: Hold the smoldering sage bundle in one hand and use the other hand to guide the smoke around the area, person, or object you want to cleanse. Start at the entrance of the space or the person's body and move the smoke in a clockwise direction, moving slowly and deliberately.

Focus on Specific Areas: Pay special attention to corners, doorways, and areas with stagnant energy. If smudging a person, move the smoke over their head, front, back, and all around them.

Use Your Intuition: Trust your intuition and take as much time as you need in each area. Visualize the negative energy being replaced by positive, pure energy.

Extinguish the Sage: Once you've smudged the entire space or object, gently extinguish the sage by pressing the burning end into the heat-resistant bowl or shell. Ensure it is completely out.

Complete the Ceremony: Express gratitude for the cleansing and purifying process. You can say a prayer or affirmation that aligns with your intention.

Why People Smudge:

People smudge for various reasons, including:

Energy Cleansing: To remove negative or stagnant energy from a space, person, or object.

Spiritual or Ritual Practices: As part of spiritual ceremonies, rituals, or meditation practices.

Aromatherapy: For the pleasant scent and calming effect of the herbs used in smudging.

Setting Intentions: To set positive intentions and create a sacred space.

Smudging Recipe with Lavender and Sage:

This smudging blend combines the purifying qualities of sage with the calming and soothing properties of lavender.

Ingredients:

1 part dried white sage

1 part dried lavender buds

Instructions:

Mix equal parts dried white sage and dried lavender buds in a bowl.

Bundle the mixture together with twine or place it in a small cloth sachet.

2. **Cedar and Sweetgrass Smudge:**

Cedar and sweetgrass are often used in Native American smudging rituals for purification and blessing. This combination offers a grounding and calming energy.

Ingredients:

Dried cedar leaves or cedar bundle

Dried sweetgrass braid

Instructions:

Bundle together a few dried cedar leaves or use a cedar bundle.

Bundle dried sweetgrass separately, making sure it's tightly braided.

Ignite the cedar bundle or leaves first, allowing it to smolder.

Once the cedar is smoldering, use the sweetgrass braid to fan the smoke and spread its purifying energy.

Use the combined smoke for smudging as you normally would.

3. **Lavender and Rose Petal Smudge:**

Lavender and rose petals create a beautiful and fragrant smudge that promotes relaxation, love, and positive energy.

Ingredients:

Dried lavender buds

Dried rose petals

Instructions:

Combine dried lavender buds and dried rose petals in equal parts.

Bundle the mixture together with twine or place it in a small cloth sachet.

Ignite the smudge and allow it to smolder.

Use the fragrant smoke to cleanse and purify your space or as a calming and loving smudge for personal use.

These additional smudging recipes offer different aromatic experiences and energies to enhance your smudging rituals. Remember to set your intention before smudging and handle smudging materials with care to ensure a safe and effective ceremony.

Chapter 4: The Alchemy of Healing: Crafting Herbal Remedies

In the heart of my grandmother's cottage, where the warmth of the kitchen stove met the fragrance of drying herbs, I found myself immersed in a world of transformation. It was a world where dried leaves, roots, and flowers became potent potions, where the ancient alchemy of healing unfolded in the skilled hands of my grandmother.

As I entered the kitchen one crisp morning, the sight that greeted me was nothing short of magical. My grandmother stood at the wooden table, surrounded by an array of glass jars, bowls of dried herbs, and a collection of gleaming copper utensils. Her hands moved with a grace that was both deliberate and intuitive, as if she were orchestrating a symphony of nature's gifts.

"Today," she announced with a twinkle in her eye, "we shall explore the art of crafting herbal remedies—potions and elixirs that carry the healing essence of the plants."

I watched in fascination as she selected a handful of dried elderberries from a jar and placed them into a copper pot. The elderberries were dark and plump, like tiny jewels glistening in the morning light.

"Elderberries," she explained, "are a powerful ally in bolstering the immune system and warding off illness. They are nature's gift to us during the cold winter months."

My grandmother poured spring water into the pot, the liquid glistening as it surrounded the elderberries. She then placed the pot on the stove and began to gently heat the mixture. As the water warmed, the elderberries released their essence, filling the kitchen with a deep, earthy aroma.

"Making herbal remedies," she said, "is a dance of patience and intention. We must allow the herbs to infuse the water with their healing energy, just as the sun infuses the earth with its warmth."

As the elderberry infusion simmered, my grandmother turned her attention to a collection of dried echinacea root. She carefully measured out a portion and added it to the pot, explaining that echinacea was a powerful immune booster that worked in harmony with elderberries.

"Herbal alchemy," she continued, "is the art of combining herbs in a way that enhances their healing properties. It is about creating synergies that amplify the effectiveness of each plant."

As we waited for the infusion to complete, my grandmother shared stories of the herbalists and healers who had mastered the craft of herbal alchemy. These wise individuals had understood the unique qualities of each plant and had learned to combine them in ways that addressed a wide range of health concerns.

"Herbalism," she said, "is not a one-size-fits-all approach. It is a practice of tailoring remedies to the individual's needs, taking into account their constitution, symptoms, and the energetics of the herbs."

Once the elderberry and echinacea infusion had simmered to perfection, my grandmother carefully strained it into a glass jar. The liquid was a rich, purplish hue—the essence of vitality captured in a simple jar.

"Infusions," she explained, "are a versatile way of extracting the healing properties of herbs. They can be consumed as teas, added to baths, or used as a base for other remedies."

With the elderberry and echinacea infusion complete, my grandmother turned her attention to another herbal ally—calendula. She selected a jar of dried calendula blossoms and placed them in a bowl.

"Calendula," she said, "is not only a healer of the body but also a balm for the skin. Its golden petals hold the secret to soothing and nourishing the skin."

My grandmother poured a carrier oil—olive oil—
into the bowl with the calendula blossoms, creating
a fragrant infusion. She explained that this
infusion would become the base for a soothing
calendula salve, a remedy that had been treasured
for centuries for its skin-healing properties.

As she worked, I couldn't help but be struck by
the simplicity of the ingredients—a few dried
herbs, some water, and a carrier oil. Yet, in her
hands, they were transformed into remedies that
held the potential to heal and nurture.

"Herbal remedies," my grandmother said, "remind
us of the profound wisdom of nature. They show us
that healing can often be found in the simplest and
most humble of ingredients."

Once the calendula infusion had steeped for
several hours, my grandmother strained it into a
clean glass jar, leaving behind the vibrant orange
petals. The liquid was infused with the healing

properties of the calendula, ready to be transformed into a salve.

She added beeswax to the calendula-infused oil and gently heated the mixture until the beeswax melted and blended with the oil. The kitchen was filled with the sweet, warm scent of beeswax, and I watched in fascination as the liquid transformed into a creamy salve.

"Beeswax," she explained, "is not only a natural emulsifier but also a protector of the skin. It creates a barrier that locks in moisture and prevents dryness."

As the calendula salve cooled and solidified, my grandmother poured it into small glass jars, labeling each one with a handwritten note indicating its contents and the date of preparation.

"Labeling," she emphasized, "is a practice of integrity and safety. It ensures that we can identify our remedies accurately and know when they were made."

The calendula salve was a tangible testament to the alchemy of healing—a transformation from dried petals to soothing balm. It was a reminder that the power to heal was not reserved for the few but was accessible to all who sought it.

In the weeks that followed, my grandmother continued to guide me through the art of crafting herbal remedies. We created tinctures from vibrant dandelion roots, brewed aromatic teas from fragrant mint leaves, and blended healing balms from comfrey and lavender. Each remedy was a testament to the versatility and potency of nature's gifts.

One particularly memorable day, my grandmother introduced me to the world of herbal teas. We ventured into the garden, where she showed me how to harvest fresh peppermint leaves. The leaves were tender and aromatic, their scent invigorating and soothing at the same time.

"Peppermint," she said, "is a plant of awakening and clarity. Its vibrant leaves carry the energy of freshness and renewal."

We carefully plucked the mint leaves and returned to the kitchen, where my grandmother set a pot of water to boil. She explained that brewing herbal teas was a practice of both science and intuition—an art that required the right proportions of herbs, the correct water temperature, and an understanding of the desired effects.

"Tea-making," she said, "is an act of mindfulness. It invites us to be fully present in the moment, to engage all our senses, and to honor the plants that grace our cups."

As the water reached a gentle boil, my grandmother placed a handful of fresh mint leaves into a teapot and poured the hot water over them. The steam rose, carrying with it the essence of mint. We let the tea steep, allowing the mint leaves to release their invigorating flavor.

"Herbal teas," my grandmother explained, "are a wonderful way to connect with the plants on a daily basis. They offer not only physical benefits but also the comfort of ritual and the joy of savoring nature's flavors."

We poured the mint tea into delicate porcelain cups and sat at the kitchen table, steam rising from our cups like a fragrant veil. As we sipped the revitalizing infusion, my grandmother shared stories of the healing traditions associated with mint—how it had been used for centuries to soothe digestive woes, alleviate headaches, and clear the mind.

"Mint tea," she said, "is a reminder of the power of simplicity. It teaches us that healing can often be found in the everyday herbs that grace our gardens."

The herbal remedies we crafted together became a tangible expression of the wisdom that my grandmother had passed down to me. They were more than mere concoctions; they were bridges to the natural world, carriers of healing energy, and testaments to the enduring magic of herbalism.

In those moments, as I watched the transformation of plants into remedies, I realized that herbalism was not just a collection of knowledge—it was a way of life, a philosophy, and a deep, abiding connection with the earth. It was a reminder that healing was not a distant concept but an intimate dance with the plants that surrounded us, a partnership with nature that was both ancient and eternal.

As I look back on those days in my grandmother's kitchen, I am filled with gratitude for the lessons she shared, for the wisdom she imparted, and for the legacy of herbalism that she entrusted to me. It was a legacy that transcended time and space, a bond that connected me to generations past and to the future generations that would carry forward the torch of healing, reverence, and the enduring magic of nature.

The alchemy of healing, as I had come to understand it, was not the stuff of fairy tales and wizardry—it was a living, breathing reality, a testament to the power of nature's gifts, and a journey of transformation that extended far beyond the confines of my grandmother's cottage. It was a journey that would shape my path, guide my choices, and infuse every aspect of my life with the profound knowledge that healing was not only possible but also a sacred art that celebrated the interconnectedness of all living beings.

1. Rosemary-Infused Olive Oil

Ingredients:

Fresh rosemary sprigs

Extra virgin olive oil

Instructions:

Collect fresh rosemary sprigs from your garden.

Place them in a clean glass jar.

Pour extra virgin olive oil over the rosemary.

Seal the jar and let it infuse for at least two weeks.

Use this aromatic oil for cooking and as a massage oil.

Words of Wisdom: "Child, just as rosemary adds flavor to meals and soothes the senses, remember that even the simplest moments can bring joy and comfort."

2. Lavender and Honey Face Mask

Ingredients:

Fresh lavender flowers

Raw honey

Instructions:

Harvest fresh lavender flowers from your garden.

Mix the lavender flowers with raw honey to create a paste.

Apply the mask to your face and leave it on for 15-20 minutes.

Rinse with warm water for refreshed and glowing skin.

Words of Wisdom: "Like the soothing touch of lavender, remember to take time for self-care and embrace your inner beauty."

3. **Basil Pesto with Garden Greens**

Ingredients:

Fresh basil leaves

Garden greens (arugula, spinach)

Garlic cloves

Pine nuts

Olive oil

Parmesan cheese (optional)

Instructions:

Harvest fresh basil and garden greens.

Blend basil, garden greens, garlic, pine nuts, and olive oil.

Add Parmesan cheese if desired.

Serve as a pasta sauce, on bread, or as a dip.

Words of Wisdom: "Much like the vibrant flavors of basil, may your life be filled with zest and enthusiasm."

4. Sage and Lemon Infused Water

Ingredients:

Fresh sage leaves

Lemon slices

Water

Instructions:

Pluck fresh sage leaves from your garden.

Place the sage leaves and lemon slices in a pitcher of water.

Let it infuse for a few hours or overnight.

Enjoy this refreshing herbal water.

Words of Wisdom: "Child, like the purity of water, may you always find clarity and renewal in life."

5. Healing Calendula Salve

Ingredients:

Fresh calendula petals

Olive oil

Beeswax

Instructions:

Gather fresh calendula petals from your garden.

Place the petals in a glass jar and cover with olive oil.

Let it sit in a sunny spot for 2-4 weeks.

Strain the infused oil and mix with melted beeswax to create a healing salve.

Apply to minor cuts, burns, or dry skin.

Words of Wisdom: "Just as calendula blooms in your garden, remember that you too have the power to heal and nurture."

6. Lemon Balm and Chamomile Tea

Ingredients:

Fresh lemon balm leaves

Chamomile flowers

Boiling water

Instructions:

Harvest fresh lemon balm leaves and chamomile flowers from your garden.

Place the leaves and flowers in a teapot.

Pour boiling water over them and steep for 5-7 minutes.

Sip this soothing tea for relaxation and calm.

Words of Wisdom: "Child, like the tranquility of this tea, may you find peace and serenity in life's moments."

7. Garden Sage Smudge Stick

Ingredients:

Fresh sage leaves

String or twine

Instructions:

Gather fresh sage leaves from your garden.

Bundle the leaves together and tie them with string or twine.

Dry the bundle in a cool, dark place until it's ready for use.

Use it for smudging and purifying your space.

Words of Wisdom: "Much like the cleansing power of sage, let go of negativity and embrace the positive energy around you."

8. Garden Mint and Strawberry Salad

Ingredients:

Fresh garden mint leaves

Fresh strawberries, sliced

Mixed salad greens

Balsamic vinaigrette dressing

Instructions:

Harvest fresh garden mint leaves, strawberries, and salad greens from your garden.

Toss them together and drizzle with balsamic vinaigrette.

Enjoy this refreshing salad.

Words of Wisdom: "Child, just as the garden mint adds a burst of freshness to the salad, may you bring vitality and joy to the world."

9. Thyme-Infused Honey

Ingredients:

Fresh thyme sprigs

Honey

Instructions:

Gather fresh thyme sprigs from your garden.

Place them in a glass jar and cover with honey.

Let it infuse for several weeks.

Use the thyme-infused honey to sweeten tea or drizzle over desserts.

Words of Wisdom: "Like the thyme in this jar, may your life be seasoned with love and warmth."

10. **Words of Wisdom**

As my grandmother would lovingly remind me:

"Dear one, a garden is not just a place of beauty;
it's a teacher of life's lessons. Just as you nurture
these herbs, remember to nurture your own spirit.
Each day is a chance to grow, bloom, and share
your unique gifts with the world. Embrace the
journey, and may your heart be as full as a
bountiful garden."

With each recipe and each moment you spend
"From Garden to Table," may you find nourishment
for your body and soul. The garden holds the
wisdom of generations, and it's a gift that keeps
on giving.

Elderberry and Echinacea Infusion

Ingredients:

1/2 cup dried elderberries

1/4 cup dried echinacea root or leaves

4 cups water

Honey (optional, for sweetness)

Instructions:

Prepare Your Workspace:

Ensure that your workspace is clean and free of contaminants. Wash your hands thoroughly.

Gather the Herbs:

Measure 1/2 cup of dried elderberries and 1/4 cup of dried echinacea root or leaves. You can adjust the quantities based on your preference and the size of your glass jar.

Boil Water:

In a medium-sized pot, bring 4 cups of water to a boil. Use filtered or distilled water for the best quality infusion.

Combine Herbs and Water:

Once the water reaches a rolling boil, carefully add the dried elderberries and echinacea to the pot.

Simmer:

Reduce the heat to low, cover the pot with a lid, and let the herbs simmer gently for about 20-30 minutes. This simmering process allows the herbs to release their beneficial compounds into the water.

Monitor the Infusion:

Keep an eye on the infusion, ensuring that it doesn't boil over. Stir occasionally to help the herbs infuse evenly.

Strain the Infusion:

After simmering, remove the pot from heat. Let it cool for a few minutes to avoid scalding yourself.

Carefully strain the hot liquid into a glass jar using a fine-mesh strainer or cheesecloth to remove all the herbs. You should be left with a rich, purplish-hued liquid—the essence of vitality captured in a simple jar.

Optional: Sweeten with Honey:

If desired, add honey to the infusion for sweetness and added health benefits. Start with a tablespoon of honey and adjust to taste. Stir until the honey is fully dissolved.

Cool and Store:

Allow the infused liquid to cool to room temperature before sealing the glass jar with a lid.

Store the infusion in the refrigerator for longer shelf life. Properly stored, it can last for several weeks.

Usage:

Consume 1-2 tablespoons of the Elderberry and Echinacea Infusion daily during cold and flu season or as a natural immune booster. You can take it straight or dilute it in water or herbal tea.

This Elderberry and Echinacea Infusion is a wonderful way to harness the immune-boosting properties of these herbs. Remember to consult with a healthcare professional if you have any underlying health conditions or are taking medications, as herbal remedies may interact with certain medications.

Calendula Salve

Ingredients:

1 cup dried calendula flowers

1 1/2 cups carrier oil (such as olive oil or coconut oil)

1/4 cup beeswax pellets or grated beeswax

A few drops of lavender essential oil (optional, for fragrance)

Instructions:

Prepare Your Workspace:

Ensure that your workspace is clean and well-ventilated. Wash your hands thoroughly and have all your ingredients and equipment ready.

Infuse the Calendula:

Place the dried calendula flowers in a clean, dry glass jar.

Heat the carrier oil (olive oil or coconut oil) in a double boiler or a heatproof glass bowl over a pot of simmering water. Heat the oil gently on low heat, but do not let it boil.

Pour the warm oil over the calendula flowers in the glass jar, making sure they are fully submerged in the oil.

Seal the jar with an airtight lid.

Infusion Process:

Allow the calendula flowers to infuse in the oil for at least 4-6 weeks. Place the jar in a cool, dark place, and shake it gently every few days to encourage infusion.

Strain the Infused Oil:

After the infusion period, strain the oil through a fine-mesh strainer or cheesecloth into a clean bowl or measuring cup. Squeeze the cloth or strainer to extract as much infused oil as possible.

Prepare Beeswax:

In a clean, dry saucepan, melt the beeswax pellets or grated beeswax over low heat. Stir gently until fully melted.

Combine Infused Oil and Beeswax:

Pour the infused calendula oil into the melted beeswax in the saucepan. Stir well to combine.

Optional: Add Lavender Essential Oil:

If you desire a fragrant salve, add a few drops of lavender essential oil to the mixture. Stir thoroughly to distribute the fragrance evenly.

Pour into Containers:

Carefully pour the warm calendula salve mixture into clean, dry containers, such as small tins or glass jars. Leave some room at the top as it will solidify upon cooling.

Cool and Solidify:

Allow the containers to cool at room temperature. The salve will solidify as it cools, forming a soothing balm.

Label and Store:

Once the calendula salve has completely solidified, label the containers with the date and contents.

Store your calendula salve in a cool, dark place. Properly stored, it can last for several months to a year.

Usage: Apply your homemade calendula salve to dry or irritated skin, minor cuts, scrapes, insect bites, or dry lips as needed. This soothing salve is a testament to the alchemy of healing, transforming dried petals into a powerful and accessible healing balm.

Chapter 5: Healing the Body and Soul: Herbal Remedies for Common Ailments

In the heart of the cottage, where the scents of dried herbs mingled with the warmth of a crackling fire, my grandmother and I embarked on a journey of healing. It was a journey that took us deep into the world of herbal remedies—a world where the plants that surrounded us held the keys to wellness, balance, and the restoration of both body and soul.

As I sat beside my grandmother one evening, the flickering candlelight casting dancing shadows on the walls, she turned to me with a gentle smile and said, "Tonight, my dear, we shall explore the realm of herbal remedies for common ailments—ailments that touch the lives of many and for which nature provides potent solutions."

I leaned in closer, eager to learn from the wellspring of knowledge that she possessed. The herbal remedies she was about to share were not just potions and elixirs; they were the embodiment of centuries of wisdom, a testament to the power of plants, and a bridge between the mundane and the miraculous.

"Let us begin," she said, her voice a soothing melody, "with a remedy that soothes the spirit and eases the burdens of the mind."

With those words, she retrieved a small jar from the medicine cabinet and placed it on the table before me. Inside the jar was a collection of dried lavender flowers, their delicate purple petals a testament to the herb's calming properties.

"Lavender," my grandmother explained, "is a beloved herb known for its ability to calm the mind and uplift the spirit. It is a remedy for the modern malady of stress and anxiety."

She instructed me to bring a kettle of water to a boil, and as the steam rose, we carefully poured the hot water over a heaping teaspoon of dried lavender flowers in a teapot. The aroma that filled the room was nothing short of enchanting—a fragrance that seemed to transport us to fields of lavender in full bloom.

"Creating an herbal infusion," my grandmother said, "is an act of mindfulness. It allows us to connect with the essence of the plant and infuse our spirits with its healing energy."

As we sipped the lavender infusion, the soothing warmth of the tea seemed to melt away the tension that had settled in my shoulders. My grandmother shared stories of lavender's ancient use in aromatherapy and herbal medicine—how it had been employed to alleviate insomnia, anxiety, and even headaches.

"Lavender," she continued, "is a reminder that even in the midst of life's chaos, there is a sanctuary of tranquility within us. It teaches us to find solace in simplicity and to embrace the healing power of nature's gifts."

With the lavender infusion still warming our souls, my grandmother turned her attention to another remedy—one that addressed the common discomfort of indigestion.

"Peppermint," she said, "is a herb with a long history of soothing digestive woes. Its vibrant leaves carry the energy of freshness and renewal."

She retrieved a jar of dried peppermint leaves from the cabinet and proceeded to brew a peppermint tea. The aroma of peppermint filled the air, invigorating and refreshing.

"Peppermint tea," my grandmother explained, "is a gentle but potent remedy for indigestion, bloating, and nausea. It helps to relax the muscles of the digestive tract and ease discomfort."

As we sipped the peppermint tea, I could feel its soothing effects—a sense of calm settling over my stomach and a renewed sense of vitality. My grandmother shared stories of how peppermint had been used by healers throughout history to alleviate a range of digestive issues.

"Herbal remedies," she said, "offer us a path to harmony and balance. They remind us that healing is not just a matter of alleviating physical symptoms but also of nurturing the spirit and restoring equilibrium."

Our exploration of herbal remedies continued, with my grandmother sharing her wisdom on how to use herbs to address a variety of common ailments. We learned about the soothing qualities of chamomile for insomnia and anxiety, the immune-boosting properties of elderberry for colds and flu, and the pain-relieving potential of willow bark for headaches and inflammation.

With each remedy, my grandmother emphasized the importance of listening to the body and approaching healing with intention and reverence. She explained that the plants we worked with were not just ingredients but living beings with their own wisdom and energy.

"Herbs," she said, "invite us into a sacred partnership with the natural world. They teach us to respect the earth's gifts and to honor the interconnectedness of all living beings."

As we delved deeper into the world of herbal remedies, I realized that the healing power of nature was vast and multifaceted. Each plant had its unique gifts, and the art of herbalism lay in understanding how to harness those gifts to restore balance and well-being.

One particularly memorable day, my grandmother introduced me to the world of herbal salves—ointments crafted from infused oils and beeswax that provided relief for various skin conditions. She had prepared a salve using comfrey and lavender, explaining that comfrey was known for its ability to promote tissue repair and reduce inflammation, while lavender added a soothing and antimicrobial quality.

"Salve-making," my grandmother said, "is a beautiful fusion of herbalism and craftsmanship. It allows us to transform herbs into topical remedies that can nourish and heal the skin."

She carefully melted beeswax and comfrey-infused oil over a gentle heat, stirring the mixture until it reached the perfect consistency. The scent of lavender mingled with the earthy aroma of comfrey, creating a fragrance that was both grounding and comforting.

"Applying herbal salves," my grandmother explained, "is a practice of self-care and self-nurturing. It reminds us to honor our bodies and to tend to our skin—the outer manifestation of our inner well-being."

As the comfrey and lavender salve cooled and solidified, my grandmother poured it into small glass jars, labeling each one with a handwritten note indicating its contents and the date of preparation. The salve was a tangible embodiment of the healing potential that lay within the plants—ready to soothe and nurture, to heal and restore.

Our journey through the world of herbal remedies continued, touching on remedies for allergies, sleeplessness, and skin irritations. My grandmother's teachings were not just about the remedies themselves but also about the philosophy of herbalism—a philosophy that celebrated the connection between humans and the natural world, a recognition of the body's innate wisdom, and a reverence for the healing potential that resided in the earth's bounty.

As I look back on those moments of discovery and learning in my grandmother's cottage, I am filled with gratitude for the profound wisdom she shared, for the knowledge that has become an integral part of my life, and for the enduring magic of herbalism. It is a world where healing is not just a matter of alleviating symptoms but a journey of connecting with the wisdom of the plants, nurturing the spirit, and restoring balance to both body and soul.

The herbal remedies my grandmother introduced me to have become more than just tools for physical well-being; they are a reminder of the profound interconnectedness of all living beings and a testament to the enduring wisdom of nature. They are a bridge that connects us to the healing energy of the earth, a reminder that the power to heal is not just a matter of science and medicine but a sacred art that celebrates the beauty, wonder, and magic of the natural world.

1. Enchanted Moonlight Elixir

Ingredients:

1 tablespoon dried rose petals

1 tablespoon dried jasmine flowers

1 teaspoon dried lavender

A pinch of dried mint

Honey to taste

Boiling water

Instructions:

In a teapot, combine rose petals, jasmine flowers, lavender, and mint.

Pour boiling water over the herbs and let steep for 10-15 minutes.

Sweeten with honey to your liking.

Sip this elixir under the moonlight to connect with your inner wisdom and intuition.

Words of Wisdom: "Child, just as the moon guides the tides, let your inner light guide your path with grace and intuition."

2. Mystical Dreamer's Tea

Ingredients:

1 tablespoon dried mugwort

1 teaspoon dried valerian root

1 teaspoon chamomile flowers

1 teaspoon dried lemon balm

A pinch of dried lavender

Boiling water

Instructions:

In a teapot, blend mugwort, valerian root, chamomile, lemon balm, and lavender.

Pour boiling water over the herbs and steep for 10 minutes.

Strain and sip before bedtime for vivid dreams and restful sleep.

Words of Wisdom: "Child, in your dreams, you may find messages from the universe. Embrace them with an open heart."

3. **Prosperity Potion**

Ingredients:

1 cinnamon stick

3 whole cloves

1 star anise

1 dried orange peel

A pinch of dried ginger

Honey to taste

Boiling water

Instructions:

In a teapot, combine cinnamon stick, cloves, star anise, orange peel, and ginger.

Pour boiling water over the spices and let steep for 5-7 minutes.

Sweeten with honey and drink to manifest prosperity and abundance.

Words of Wisdom: "Child, as you sip this potion, remember that abundance flows to those with a grateful heart."

4. Elemental Harmony Elixir

Ingredients:

1 tablespoon dried nettle leaves

1 tablespoon dried chamomile flowers

1 teaspoon dried sage leaves

A pinch of dried mint

Honey to taste

Boiling water

Instructions:

In a teapot, blend nettle leaves, chamomile flowers, sage leaves, and mint.

Pour boiling water over the herbs and steep for 10 minutes.

Sweeten with honey and savor to restore balance and harmony.

Words of Wisdom: "Child, like the elements, you too have the power to find balance within yourself and your surroundings."

5. Heart's Ease Tincture

Ingredients:

Fresh hawthorn berries

Fresh rose petals

Brandy or vodka

Instructions:

Gather hawthorn berries and rose petals.

Place them in a glass jar and cover with brandy or vodka.

Let it steep for at least six weeks.

Strain and take a few drops daily to nourish your heart and spirit.

Words of Wisdom: "Much like the heart's ease tincture, let your heart bloom with love and compassion."

6. Earth's Embrace Bath Salts

Ingredients:

Epsom salt

Dried lavender flowers

Dried rosemary

A few drops of cedarwood essential oil

Instructions:

Mix Epsom salt, dried lavender flowers, and dried rosemary in a bowl.

Add a few drops of cedarwood essential oil.

Sprinkle these bath salts into your warm bath for grounding and relaxation.

Words of Wisdom: "Child, just as you immerse yourself in this soothing bath, immerse your soul in the beauty of the natural world."

7. **Dragon's Breath Fire Cider**

Ingredients:

1 cup apple cider vinegar

1/4 cup chopped fresh horseradish

1/4 cup chopped fresh ginger

1/4 cup chopped fresh garlic

1/4 cup chopped fresh onion

A pinch of cayenne pepper

A pinch of turmeric powder

Instructions:

Combine apple cider vinegar, horseradish, ginger, garlic, onion, cayenne pepper, and turmeric in a glass jar.

Seal the jar and let it sit in a dark place for 2-4 weeks.

Strain and take a tablespoon daily for immune support and vitality.

Words of Wisdom: "Child, just as the dragon's breath ignites passion, may your spirit burn bright with determination and courage."

8. Luna's Blessing Incense

Ingredients:

Dried frankincense resin

Dried myrrh resin

Dried mugwort

Dried lavender flowers

Instructions:

Combine dried frankincense, myrrh, mugwort, and lavender in a mortar and pestle.

Grind into a fine powder.

Burn this incense during lunar rituals for blessings and protection.

Words of Wisdom: "Like the incense's aroma, let the energy of your intentions rise and permeate the universe."

9. Guardian of the Forest Balm

Ingredients:

Fresh pine resin

Beeswax

Olive oil

Instructions:

Collect fresh pine resin from the forest.

Melt beeswax in a double boiler.

Add pine resin and olive oil to create a healing balm.

Use it on minor cuts, insect bites, or as a protective salve.

Words of Wisdom: "Child, like the forest's guardians, stand tall, and protect the beauty and balance of your world."

10. Words of Wisdom

As my grandmother would lovingly remind me:

"Dear one, the alchemy of blending herbs is a reflection of your inner magic. Just as you create these remedies with intention and creativity, remember that your life is a canvas, and your choices are the colors that paint your journey. Embrace your uniqueness and let your heart guide your craft."

With every blend you create and every intention you set, may you find the artistry and healing within yourself. The world is your canvas, and you are the artist of your destiny.

Chapter 6: Nurturing the Body and Soul: Herbal Remedies for Everyday Wellness

The sun bathed my grandmother's garden in a soft, golden glow as we gathered beneath the shade of an ancient oak tree. This serene setting had become our sanctuary—a place where the wisdom of generations mingled with the healing energy of nature, and where the gentle whispers of leaves carried secrets of herbal remedies for everyday wellness.

My grandmother turned to me with a knowing smile and said, "Today, my dear, we shall delve deeper into the world of herbal remedies. These are not just potions and elixirs; they are the keys to nurturing our bodies and souls, helping us maintain balance and vitality in the ebb and flow of everyday life."

I leaned in closer, eager to uncover the treasures of knowledge she had to share. The remedies we were about to explore were more than just solutions for common ailments—they were the embodiment of holistic well-being, a celebration of the interplay between the physical and spiritual aspects of our existence.

"Let us begin," she said, "with a remedy that nourishes the body and soothes the soul."

With those words, my grandmother led me to a flourishing patch of lemon balm. The leaves of this fragrant herb glistened with dewdrops, releasing a citrusy aroma that danced on the breeze.

"Lemon balm," she explained, "is a herb of joy and renewal. Its vibrant leaves carry the energy of sunshine and can help alleviate stress, anxiety, and even mild depression."

We carefully harvested a handful of lemon balm leaves and returned to the kitchen, where my grandmother set a kettle of water to boil. As the steam rose, we placed the fresh leaves into a teapot and poured the hot water over them, allowing the lemon balm to infuse the liquid with its bright essence.

"Brewing herbal teas," my grandmother said, "is a practice of both science and intuition. It's about the right proportions, the correct water temperature, and understanding the desired effects of the remedy."

We sipped the lemon balm tea, its gentle citrus notes offering both comfort and a sense of renewal. My grandmother shared stories of how lemon balm had been used for centuries to promote relaxation, improve mood, and uplift the spirit.

"Lemon balm," she continued, "reminds us that wellness is not just the absence of illness but a state of joy, balance, and contentment. It teaches us to find solace in simplicity and to embrace the healing power of nature's gifts."

With the lemon balm tea still warming our hearts, my grandmother turned her attention to a remedy that addressed the common discomfort of indigestion.

"Ginger," she said, "is a root with a long history of soothing digestive woes. Its warming qualities can alleviate nausea, bloating, and indigestion."

She retrieved a piece of fresh ginger root from the pantry and showed me how to prepare ginger tea. We sliced the ginger into thin rounds and simmered them in hot water until the liquid became infused with the root's spicy warmth.

"Ginger tea," my grandmother explained, "is a remedy that not only soothes the stomach but also invigorates the senses. It awakens the body and the spirit."

We sipped the ginger tea, its spicy notes tingling on our tongues and bringing a sense of vitality. My grandmother shared stories of how ginger had been used as a digestive aid and a remedy for motion sickness and morning sickness.

"Herbal remedies," she said, "offer us a holistic approach to well-being. They remind us that our physical health is intimately connected to our emotional and spiritual states."

Our exploration of herbal remedies continued, with my grandmother imparting her wisdom on how to use herbs to nurture the body and soul. We learned about the calming qualities of chamomile for stress and anxiety, the immune-boosting properties of echinacea for colds and flu, and the rejuvenating potential of nettle for energy and vitality.

With each remedy, my grandmother emphasized the importance of mindfulness and intention. She explained that the plants we worked with were not just ingredients but living beings with their own wisdom and energy.

"Herbs," she said, "invite us into a sacred partnership with the natural world. They teach us to respect the earth's gifts and to honor the interconnectedness of all living beings."

As we delved deeper into the world of herbal remedies, I realized that they were not just tools for physical well-being but gateways to a deeper understanding of our own inner landscapes. They offered a path to balance and harmony, a reminder that wellness was not just a matter of alleviating physical symptoms but also of nurturing the spirit and restoring equilibrium.

One particularly memorable day, my grandmother introduced me to the world of herbal baths—an ancient practice of immersing oneself in the healing energies of herbs and flowers. We ventured into the garden, where she showed me how to harvest fragrant rose petals and lavender blossoms.

"Herbal baths," my grandmother said, "are a luxurious and soul-nourishing way to connect with the plants. They offer relaxation for the body and a deep sense of well-being for the spirit."

We filled a large basin with warm water and added the rose petals and lavender blossoms. The scent that rose from the water was nothing short of enchanting—a fragrance that seemed to transport us to fields of blooming flowers.

As I eased into the herbal bath, the warm water embraced me, and the aromatic steam enveloped my senses. It was a moment of profound relaxation, a retreat from the hustle and bustle of everyday life.

"Herbal baths," my grandmother continued, "are a reminder that self-care is not a luxury but a necessity. They invite us to honor our bodies, to release tension, and to nurture the soul."

Our journey through the world of herbal remedies expanded to include remedies for allergies, sleeplessness, and skin irritations. My grandmother's teachings were not just about the remedies themselves but also about the philosophy of herbalism—a philosophy that celebrated the connection between humans and the natural world, a recognition of the body's innate wisdom, and a reverence for the healing potential that resided in the earth's bounty.

As I look back on those moments of discovery and learning in my grandmother's cottage, I am filled with gratitude for the profound wisdom she shared, for the knowledge that has become an integral part of my life, and for the enduring magic of herbalism. It is a world where healing is not just a matter of alleviating symptoms but a journey of connecting with the wisdom of the plants, nurturing the spirit, and restoring balance to both body and soul.

Our exploration of herbal remedies became a tapestry of well-being—a celebration of the interconnectedness of all living beings, the wisdom of the plants, and the enduring magic of the earth. It was a reminder that healing was not just a matter of science and medicine but a sacred art that celebrated the beauty, wonder, and interconnectedness of the natural world.

In the heart of my grandmother's garden, I discovered not only the tools of herbalism but also the essence of healing—a journey that extended beyond the confines of the garden and into the very heart of nature itself. It was a journey that celebrated the interplay between the physical and spiritual aspects of our existence, a recognition of our place in the web of life, and a deep reverence for the healing potential that resided within us and all around us.

1. Serenity Sipper Tea

Ingredients:

1 tablespoon dried lemon balm

1 tablespoon dried chamomile flowers

1 teaspoon dried lavender

1 teaspoon dried rose petals

Honey to taste

Boiling water

Instructions:

In a teapot, combine lemon balm, chamomile, lavender, and rose petals.

Pour boiling water over the herbs and let steep for 10-15 minutes.

Sweeten with honey to your liking.

Sip this soothing tea to find serenity and peace within.

Words of Wisdom: "Child, as you sip this tea, remember that inner peace is a treasure that blooms within your heart."

2. Inner Harmony Elixir

Ingredients:

Fresh hawthorn berries

Fresh St. John's Wort flowers

Fresh lemon balm leaves

Brandy or vodka

Instructions:

Gather hawthorn berries, St. John's Wort flowers, and lemon balm leaves.

Place them in a glass jar and cover with brandy or vodka.

Let it steep for at least six weeks.

Take a few drops daily to restore inner harmony and emotional balance.

Words of Wisdom: "Much like the elixir, may your heart find harmony, even in life's challenging moments."

3. Joyful Blossom Bath Soak

Ingredients:

Epsom salt

Dried calendula petals

Dried orange peel

A few drops of ylang-ylang essential oil

Instructions:

Mix Epsom salt, dried calendula petals, and dried orange peel in a bowl.

Add a few drops of ylang-ylang essential oil.

Sprinkle these bath salts into your warm bath to uplift your spirits and embrace joy.

Words of Wisdom: "Child, as you soak in this bath, allow joy to fill your heart, just as these blossoms fill the air with their fragrance."

4. Heartfelt Herbal Honey

Ingredients:

Fresh rose petals

Raw honey

Instructions:

Harvest fresh rose petals from your garden.

Mix the petals with raw honey to create an infused honey.

Allow it to sit for a few weeks.

Use this heartfelt herbal honey as a sweetener or drizzle it over desserts.

Words of Wisdom: "Like the sweet embrace of honey, let love be the foundation of your life."

5. Empowerment Elixir

Ingredients:1 cinnamon stick

3 cardamom pods

1 teaspoon dried rosemary

A pinch of dried ginger

A pinch of dried cloves

Honey to taste

Boiling water

Instructions:

In a teapot, combine cinnamon stick, cardamom pods, rosemary, ginger, and cloves.

Pour boiling water over the spices and let steep for 5-7 minutes.

Sweeten with honey and drink to empower your spirit and boost self-confidence.

Words of Wisdom: "Child, as you sip this elixir, remember that your inner strength is as powerful as the spices within."

6. Tranquil Moon Elixir

Ingredients:

Fresh passionflower leaves and flowers

Fresh lemon balm leaves

Brandy or vodka

Instructions:

Gather passionflower leaves, passionflower flowers, and lemon balm leaves.

Place them in a glass jar and cover with brandy or vodka.

Let it steep for at least six weeks.

Take a few drops before bedtime to experience tranquility and restful sleep.

Words of Wisdom: "Much like the tranquil moon, may your soul find serenity in the quiet moments of the night."

7. Blissful Berry Infusion

Ingredients:

Dried elderberries

Dried hibiscus petals

Dried lavender

Boiling water

Instructions:

In a teapot, combine elderberries, hibiscus petals, and lavender.

Pour boiling water over the herbs and let steep for 10-15 minutes.

Sip this infusion to awaken feelings of bliss and contentment.

Words of Wisdom: "Child, like the blend of flavors in this infusion, may your life be a symphony of joyful moments."

8. Self-Love Spell Sachet

Ingredients:

Pink or red fabric

Rose quartz crystal

Dried rose petals

Lavender buds

Pink ribbon

Instructions:

Cut a small square of pink or red fabric.

Place a rose quartz crystal, dried rose petals, and lavender buds in the center.

Gather the corners and tie with a pink ribbon.

Carry this sachet with you as a reminder to love and care for yourself.

Words of Wisdom: "Just as you hold this sachet close, hold your self-worth and self-love even closer."

9. Moonlit Meadow Salve

Ingredients:

Fresh meadowfoam flowers

Beeswax

Olive oil

Instructions:

Collect fresh meadowfoam flowers from a moonlit meadow.

Melt beeswax in a double boiler.

Add meadowfoam flowers and olive oil to create a soothing salve.

Use it as a balm for dry skin or as a nighttime ritual to connect with the moon's energy.

Words of Wisdom: "Child, just as the moonlight bathes the meadow, may your spirit be bathed in light and tranquility."

10. Words of Wisdom

As my grandmother would lovingly remind me:

"Dear one, the herbs for the heart and soul are a reflection of the beauty within you. As you explore their magic, remember that you, too, possess the power to nurture your inner landscape. Your emotions and spirit are as important as your physical health. Embrace the herbs and remedies that resonate with your soul, and may your heart be a garden of love and joy."

With each herbal creation and each moment of self-discovery, may you find the peace, balance, and serenity that nourishes your heart and soul. Your inner world is a reflection of your outer world, so tend to it with care and love.

Creating an altar for your herbal remedies is a beautiful and meaningful practice that can enhance the energy and intention behind your remedies. It's a way to connect with the energies of the plants, acknowledge their gifts, and infuse your remedies with blessings. Here are directions on how to create such an altar, along with the words of wisdom from my grandmother:

Creating an Herbal Remedy Altar:

Materials Needed:

A small table or surface

A clean, natural cloth or scarf to cover the table (preferably in earthy tones)

Small decorative containers or dishes

Fresh or dried herbs, flowers, or plants associated with your remedies

Small crystals or stones (optional)

A small bowl of water

A candle and a lighter or matches

A handwritten or printed note with your grandmother's words of wisdom

Instructions:

Select a Location: Choose a quiet and peaceful space in your home or garden where you can set up your herbal remedy altar. It should be a place where you can sit or stand comfortably and connect with the energies of nature.

Prepare the Table: Place the clean, natural cloth or scarf on the table or surface. This represents the earth element and provides a serene foundation for your altar.

Arrange the Elements: On the cloth, arrange the small containers or dishes. These will serve as vessels for your herbs and other elements. You can place them in a way that feels harmonious to you.

Add the Herbs: Select the herbs, flowers, or plants associated with the remedies you've created. These can be fresh or dried, depending on your preference and what's available. Place them in the containers or dishes, arranging them with care.

Incorporate Crystals (Optional): If you work with crystals or stones, you can add small ones to your altar. Choose crystals that resonate with the energy of healing and intention. Place them near the herbs or in a separate container.

Include a Bowl of Water: Water symbolizes the element of water, which represents emotions and intuition. Place a small bowl of water on the altar, either next to the herbs or in a central position.

Light a Candle: Place a candle on the altar and light it. Fire symbolizes transformation and the element of fire. It also adds a beautiful and sacred ambiance to your altar.

Display Your Words of Wisdom: Take the handwritten or printed note with your grandmother's words of wisdom and place it on the altar. This note serves as a reminder of the intention and purpose of your altar.

Sit in Reverence: Take a moment to sit quietly in front of your herbal remedy altar. Close your eyes, take a few deep breaths, and connect with the energy and intention you've infused into this sacred space.

Offer Gratitude: As you sit in front of your altar, offer gratitude to the plants, the earth, and the energies that support your healing journey. You can silently or verbally express your thanks.

Use the Altar: When you prepare or use your herbal remedies, do so at your altar. Infuse each remedy with blessings, intention, and love. You can also meditate, journal, or simply spend time in contemplation at your altar to deepen your connection with the healing energies.

Why Create an Herbal Remedy Altar:

Creating an herbal remedy altar serves several purposes:

Intention and Focus: It helps you set clear intentions for your herbal remedies and rituals, enhancing their effectiveness.

Connection with Nature: It deepens your connection with the energies of the plants and the natural world, honoring the gifts of the earth.

Sacred Space: It provides a dedicated and sacred space where you can perform healing rituals, meditate, or simply be in the presence of healing energy.

Mindfulness: It encourages mindfulness and gratitude, reminding you to be present and appreciative of the healing journey.

Words of Wisdom from my Grandmother:

"An altar," she said, "is a place of reverence and intention. It is a sacred space where we can connect with the energies of the plants, offer gratitude for their gifts, and infuse our remedies with blessings."

These words of wisdom emphasize the sacredness of the herbal remedy altar and the profound connection it fosters between you, the plants, and the healing energies that flow through your remedies.

Chapter 7: Seasons of Healing: Herbal Remedies for Holistic Wellness

In my grandmother's garden, time flowed like a gentle stream, marking the passage of seasons with the rhythm of nature's heartbeat. Each season brought its own gifts, its own challenges, and its own opportunities for healing. As I stood amidst the vibrant tapestry of herbs, flowers, and trees, I realized that our journey through herbal remedies was intricately woven into the changing seasons of the natural world.

My grandmother and I had spent countless hours tending to the garden, observing the ebb and flow of life, and discovering the ways in which herbs and plants aligned with the cycles of the earth. She had taught me that the art of herbalism was not just about knowing which plants to use but also about understanding when and how to harness their healing energies.

"Today," my grandmother said with a twinkle in her eye, "we shall explore the profound connection between herbal remedies and the seasons. Nature offers us a rich tapestry of herbs, each with its unique qualities, and the changing seasons guide us in using them for holistic wellness."

As I listened intently, I realized that our journey was about to take a deeper dive into the wisdom of the earth, the intricate dance of the seasons, and the artistry of herbal remedies that harmonized with the cycles of life.

Spring: Renewal and Rejuvenation

With the arrival of spring, the garden burst into a riot of colors and fragrances. It was a time of renewal, when life awakened from its winter slumber and the earth seemed to hum with vitality. My grandmother led me to a bed of vibrant dandelion leaves and blossoms.

"Dandelion," she explained, "is a springtime gift from nature. Its bitter leaves and sunny blossoms are a tonic for the liver, helping to cleanse and rejuvenate the body after the heaviness of winter."

We carefully harvested dandelion leaves and blossoms, and my grandmother showed me how to prepare a dandelion tea. The leaves and blossoms were steeped in hot water, creating a beverage that was both refreshing and revitalizing.

"As spring awakens the earth," my grandmother said, "it also awakens our bodies. Dandelion reminds us to embrace change and release what no longer serves us, just as the earth sheds its winter cloak."

The dandelion tea carried a hint of bitterness, a reminder that renewal often required letting go of old patterns and embracing the new. As we sipped the tea, my grandmother shared stories of how dandelion had been used as a springtime tonic for centuries, promoting healthy digestion, clear skin, and a sense of lightness.

"Spring," she continued, "is a season of both physical and spiritual cleansing. It invites us to shed the layers of stagnation and welcome the energy of growth and transformation."

Summer: Abundance and Vitality

As the days grew longer and the sun bathed the garden in warmth, my grandmother and I turned our attention to the abundance of summer. It was a season of fullness, when the garden offered a cornucopia of herbs and flowers, each bursting with vitality and energy.

"Summer," my grandmother said, "is a time of nourishment and celebration. It is a season when the earth provides generously, and our bodies thrive on the gifts of nature."

We ventured to a fragrant patch of lavender in full bloom. The purple spikes swayed in the breeze, releasing their soothing aroma.

"Lavender," my grandmother explained, "is a summer ally for both body and soul. Its aromatic blossoms can calm the mind, ease tension, and promote restful sleep."

We harvested lavender blossoms and returned to the kitchen, where we prepared a lavender-infused honey. The blossoms were gently placed in a jar of honey, and over time, the honey absorbed the essence of the lavender, creating a sweet elixir of relaxation and vitality.

"Lavender-infused honey," my grandmother said, "is a reminder to savor the sweetness of life, to find moments of tranquility amid the busyness of summer, and to nurture the body and soul with the gifts of the season."

As we enjoyed a spoonful of lavender-infused honey, I felt a sense of calm wash over me, a deep connection with the rhythms of the earth, and a recognition of the importance of savoring the abundance of summer.

"Summer," my grandmother continued, "is a time to embrace the fullness of life, to nourish ourselves with the richness of the earth, and to celebrate the vitality that surrounds us."

Autumn: Harvest and Reflection

With the arrival of autumn, the garden transformed into a tapestry of golden hues and russet tones. It was a season of harvest and reflection, when the earth's bounty reached its peak, and the air was filled with a sense of gratitude for the abundance of the year.

My grandmother led me to a patch of echinacea, its vibrant purple petals a testament to its immune-boosting properties.

"Echinacea," she explained, "is an autumn warrior. Its roots and blossoms are a powerful ally in strengthening the immune system, preparing the body for the challenges of the colder months."

We carefully dug up the echinacea roots, leaving some in the ground to ensure their return in the following years. Back in the kitchen, my grandmother showed me how to create an echinacea tincture—a potent extract that would help fortify the body's defenses.

"Echinacea tincture," my grandmother said, "is a reminder to honor the cycles of life. Autumn invites us to harvest the fruits of our labor, to reflect on the lessons of the year, and to prepare for the quieter months ahead."

As we prepared the echinacea tincture, I couldn't help but feel a sense of gratitude for the wisdom of the plants and the guidance of my grandmother. The tincture would be a guardian of health throughout the winter, a reminder of the interconnectedness of all living beings, and a testament to the beauty of the changing seasons.

"Autumn," my grandmother continued, "is a season of both abundance and release. It teaches us that life is cyclical, that every ending holds the promise of a new beginning, and that we are part of a greater tapestry of existence."

Winter: Rest and Renewal

As winter descended upon the garden, the landscape transformed into a serene tableau of snow and frost. It was a season of rest and renewal, a time when the earth slumbered beneath its white blanket, and the garden awaited the promise of spring.

My grandmother led me to a quiet corner of the garden where a patch of chamomile lay dormant under the snow.

"Chamomile," she explained, "is a winter companion for inner reflection and gentle healing. Its blossoms offer a sense of calm and comfort during the cold months."

We carefully harvested dried chamomile blossoms from our stores and prepared a chamomile tea. The steam rose from the cup like a wisp of warmth on a cold winter's day.

"Chamomile tea," my grandmother said, "is a reminder to embrace the stillness of winter, to turn inward, and to nurture the spirit. It is a balm for the soul during the quieter months."

As we sipped the chamomile tea, I felt a sense of serenity envelop me—a connection with the wisdom of the season and an appreciation for the cycles of rest and renewal.

"Winter," my grandmother continued, "is a time to rest, to replenish our inner resources, and to prepare for the awakening of spring. It is a season of quietude and introspection, a reminder that healing encompasses the body, mind, and spirit."

The Dance of the Seasons

As I looked back on our journey through the seasons of healing, I realized that it was not just a lesson in herbal remedies but a profound exploration of our connection to the earth and the cycles of life. Each season had offered its unique wisdom, guiding us in nurturing our bodies and souls with the gifts of nature.

My grandmother's teachings had shown me that herbal remedies were not just about addressing physical symptoms but about harmonizing with the rhythms of the natural world, acknowledging the interconnectedness of all living beings, and finding balance and vitality in every season.

"Herbs," my grandmother said, "are our allies in the dance of the seasons. They teach us to live in harmony with the earth, to honor the wisdom of the plants, and to celebrate the ever-changing tapestry of life."

As we stood in her garden, I felt a deep sense of gratitude for the knowledge she had shared, for the wisdom of the seasons, and for the enduring magic of herbalism. It was a world where healing was not just a matter of science and medicine but a sacred art that celebrated the beauty, wonder, and interconnectedness of the natural world.

In the heart of the garden, I had discovered not only the remedies for physical well-being but also the essence of holistic healing—a journey that extended beyond the confines of the garden and into the very heart of nature itself. It was a journey that celebrated the cycles of life, the interconnectedness of all living beings, and the enduring magic of the earth.

1. **Soothing Sage and Honey Throat Lozenges**

Ingredients:

Fresh sage leaves

Raw honey

Cornstarch (optional)

Instructions:

Harvest fresh sage leaves.

Coat the leaves with raw honey.

Dust them with a light layer of cornstarch if desired.

Let them dry and harden.

Use as throat lozenges to soothe sore throats and coughs.

Words of Wisdom: "Child, just as these lozenges soothe your throat, remember that your voice holds the power to heal and comfort."

2. Digestive Bitters Tonic

Ingredients:

Dandelion root

Gentian root

Orange peel

Vodka or brandy

Instructions:

Combine dandelion root, gentian root, and orange peel in a glass jar.

Cover with vodka or brandy.

Let it steep for several weeks.

Take a few drops before meals to aid digestion.

Words of Wisdom: "Like the tonic's bitter taste, life's challenges can be transformed into opportunities for growth."

3. **Herbal Steam for Sinus Relief**

Ingredients:

Eucalyptus leaves

Peppermint leaves

Boiling water

Instructions:

Combine eucalyptus leaves and peppermint leaves in a bowl.

Pour boiling water over the herbs.

Lean over the bowl, covering your head with a towel.

Inhale the steam to relieve sinus congestion.

Words of Wisdom: "Child, just as this steam clears your sinuses, let go of negativity to find clarity within."

4. **Energizing Citrus and Ginger Bath Salts**

Ingredients:

Epsom salt

Dried lemon peel

Dried orange peel

Dried ginger powder

A few drops of grapefruit essential oil

Instructions:

Mix Epsom salt, dried lemon peel, dried orange peel, and dried ginger powder in a bowl.

Add a few drops of grapefruit essential oil.

Add these bath salts to your warm bath for an energizing soak.

Words of Wisdom: "Much like the citrus and ginger, let your spirit be invigorated by the zest of life."

5. Lavender and Rosemary Headache Balm

Ingredients:

Fresh lavender flowers

Fresh rosemary leaves

Olive oil

Beeswax

Instructions:

Collect fresh lavender flowers and rosemary leaves.

Infuse them in olive oil for several weeks.

Strain the oil and mix with melted beeswax to create a soothing balm.

Apply to your temples for headache relief.

Words of Wisdom: "Child, just as this balm eases your pain, remember that challenges too shall pass."

6. **Immune-Boosting Elderberry Gummies**

Ingredients:

Elderberry syrup

Gelatin

Instructions:

Mix elderberry syrup with gelatin in a saucepan.

Heat and stir until the mixture is smooth.

Pour into silicone molds and let them set.

Enjoy these gummies to support your immune system.

Words of Wisdom: "Like the elderberries in these gummies, may your immune system be strong and resilient."

7. **Calming Chamomile Eye Compress**

Ingredients:

Chamomile tea bags

Hot water

Instructions:

Steep chamomile tea bags in hot water.

Let them cool slightly.

Place the warm tea bags over your closed eyes for relaxation and relief from eye strain.

Words of Wisdom: "Child, as you rest your eyes with chamomile, may you find peace in moments of rest."

8. Nourishing Oatmeal Bath for Dry Skin

Ingredients:

Rolled oats

Lavender essential oil

Milk (optional)

Instructions:

Grind rolled oats into a fine powder.

Add a few drops of lavender essential oil.

Sprinkle this mixture into your warm bath for soothing dry skin.

Add milk if desired for extra nourishment.

Words of Wisdom: "Much like this bath, remember to nurture your skin and soul with self-care."

9. Anti-Anxiety Lavender and Lemon Balm Tincture

Ingredients:

Fresh lavender flowers

Fresh lemon balm leaves

Brandy or vodka

Instructions:

Gather fresh lavender flowers and lemon balm leaves.

Place them in a glass jar and cover with brandy or vodka.

Let it steep for at least six weeks.

Take a few drops when needed to ease anxiety and promote calmness.

Words of Wisdom: "Child, like the calming effect of this tincture, may you find peace within, even in life's storms."

10. **Words of Wisdom**

As my grandmother would lovingly remind me:

"Dear one, everyday ailments are part of life's journey. Just as you find remedies in nature, remember that challenges are opportunities for growth and healing. Embrace the wisdom of your own body and spirit. Trust in the power of nature to nurture and restore you."

With each remedy and each challenge you face, may you grow stronger and wiser. Life's trials are your teachers, and you have the tools to heal and thrive.

Chapter 8: The Art of Herbal Blending: Crafting Remedies with Intention

In my grandmother's garden, the air was alive with the scent of blooming herbs and the gentle hum of bees. As I walked along the winding paths, I couldn't help but marvel at the beauty and abundance that surrounded me. This garden was not just a collection of plants; it was a tapestry of healing, a sanctuary of wisdom, and a living testament to the art of herbal blending.

My grandmother had taught me that herbalism was more than just knowing individual remedies—it was about the alchemical dance of combining herbs to create potent and balanced formulations. Each blend was a work of art, a harmony of flavors and energies, and a reflection of the herbalist's intention.

"Today," my grandmother said, her eyes sparkling with anticipation, "we shall explore the art of herbal blending—a practice that invites us to craft remedies with intention and creativity."

With those words, she led me to a table set up in a quiet corner of the garden. On the table were an array of dried herbs, flowers, and spices, each carefully selected for their unique properties and energies.

"Herbal blending," my grandmother explained, "is a sacred art that honors the wisdom of the plants and the healing potential of synergy. It allows us to create remedies that address a wide range of needs, from physical ailments to emotional imbalances."

As I gazed at the colorful array before me, I realized that this was not just a lesson in herbalism—it was an invitation to become a co-creator with nature, to tap into the creative flow, and to infuse our remedies with intention and magic.

The Basics of Herbal Blending

My grandmother began our lesson by introducing me to the foundational principles of herbal blending:

1. Synergy: "When we blend herbs," she said, "we create a synergy—an interaction where the combined effect is greater than the sum of individual herbs. It's like a beautiful symphony where each instrument plays its part to create harmony."

2. Intention: "The intention behind a blend is crucial," my grandmother emphasized. "We must ask ourselves, 'What is the purpose of this remedy?' Is it to soothe, invigorate, or restore balance? Our intention infuses the blend with purpose and energy."

3. Flavor Profiling: My grandmother encouraged me to engage my senses. "Taste and aroma are essential," she explained. "We must consider how the blend will taste and smell, as these qualities

can enhance the overall experience and therapeutic effect."

4. Dosage and Safety: "Herbal blending requires an understanding of dosage and safety," she cautioned. "Some herbs are potent and require caution in their use. It's important to research each herb and its contraindications."

Armed with these principles, we began our journey into the world of herbal blending.

Balancing Act: Calming Tea Blend

Our first creation was a calming tea blend—an elixir designed to soothe frayed nerves and promote relaxation. My grandmother guided me through the selection of herbs, carefully considering their properties and energies.

We started with chamomile, a gentle herb known for its calming effects on the nervous system. Next came lemon balm, which added a touch of lemony brightness to the blend while further enhancing its soothing properties. We included a sprinkle of lavender blossoms for their aromatic beauty and relaxation-inducing qualities.

"The key to blending," my grandmother explained, "is balance. We want the flavors and energies of these herbs to complement each other, creating a harmonious and effective blend."

We mixed the dried herbs in a bowl, our hands gently cradling the fragrant mixture. As I inhaled the aroma, I felt a sense of tranquility washing over me—a preview of the calming effect this blend would have.

"Intention is important," my grandmother said as we prepared the tea. "As we steep the herbs, we infuse the blend with our intention for peace, relaxation, and inner calm. This makes the remedy not only effective but also a mindful practice of healing."

As we sipped the calming tea, I marveled at the artistry of herbal blending. The flavors danced on my tongue, the aroma enveloped my senses, and I felt a deep sense of relaxation—a testament to the power of intention and synergy.

Energizing Elixir: Morning Vitality Blend

Our next creation was an energizing elixir—a blend designed to awaken the senses and provide a boost of vitality to start the day. We selected herbs that offered a combination of invigoration and mental clarity.

We began with peppermint, a refreshing herb that awakened the senses with its cool, minty flavor. To enhance mental alertness, we added rosemary, an herb known for its cognitive benefits. Finally, a touch of lemon verbena brought a zesty brightness to the blend.

"Herbal blending," my grandmother explained, "allows us to create remedies that support not only the physical but also the mental and emotional aspects of well-being. This morning vitality blend is a testament to that."

As we mixed the dried herbs, I noticed how the colors, textures, and aromas harmonized beautifully. It was a blend that embodied the vitality of a new day, a promise of energy and clarity.

"Intention is key here as well," my grandmother said. "As we sip this elixir in the morning, we infuse it with our intention for a day filled with vitality, focus, and joy."

As I sipped the morning vitality blend, I felt a surge of energy and mental clarity—an awakening of body and spirit. It was a reminder that herbal remedies were not just about addressing physical needs but also about nourishing the soul and aligning with our intentions.

Harmony in a Bottle: Stress-Relief Tincture

Our final creation was a stress-relief tincture—a remedy designed to provide emotional balance and support during times of tension and anxiety.

We chose herbs that worked synergistically to calm the nervous system and ease emotional strain. Milky oats, with their soothing properties, formed the foundation of the tincture. To further enhance its calming effect, we added passionflower and skullcap, both known for their ability to alleviate stress and anxiety.

"The beauty of herbal blending," my grandmother said, "is that we can create remedies that address the root causes of imbalances, whether they are physical, emotional, or spiritual. This tincture is a testament to the holistic nature of herbalism."

As we prepared the tincture, my grandmother explained the importance of patience in the herbal blending process. "Tinctures require time," she said. "The herbs need time to infuse the alcohol with their healing properties. It's a reminder that healing, too, is a process that unfolds over time."

We poured the alcohol over the dried herbs, sealing the tincture jar with care. My grandmother emphasized the role of intention once more. "As this tincture matures," she said, "it will absorb our intention for peace, balance, and emotional well-being. It becomes not just a remedy but a reflection of our inner harmony."

As we concluded our lesson in herbal blending, I couldn't help but feel a deep sense of reverence for the plants, for the wisdom of my grandmother, and for the artistry of creating remedies with intention.

"Herbal blending," my grandmother said, "is a sacred practice that honors the interconnectedness of all living beings. It reminds us that we are not separate from nature but integral parts of it. When we blend with intention and respect, we become co-creators with the earth, weaving healing into every remedy we craft."

In the heart of the garden, I had learned not only the techniques of herbal blending but also the essence of healing—a journey that extended beyond the confines of the garden and into the very heart of nature itself. It was a journey of creativity, intention, and a deep reverence for the enduring magic of herbalism—a world where healing was not just a matter of science and medicine but a sacred art that celebrated the beauty, wonder, and interconnectedness of the natural world.

1. Sacred Space Herbal Smudge Bundle

Ingredients:

Fresh sage leaves

Fresh rosemary sprigs

Lavender flowers

Thin twine or string

Instructions:

Gather sage leaves, rosemary sprigs, and lavender flowers from your garden.

Bundle them together and tie with twine.

Allow the bundle to dry in a sacred space.

Use it to cleanse and purify your surroundings, inviting positive energies.

Words of Wisdom: "Child, as you cleanse with this smudge bundle, remember to purify your heart and mind."

2. **Moonlight Meditation Tea**

Ingredients:

Fresh lemon balm leaves

Fresh mint leaves

Fresh chamomile flowers

Boiling water

Instructions:

Harvest fresh lemon balm, mint, and chamomile from your garden.

Combine them in a teapot.

Pour boiling water over the herbs and steep for 10-15 minutes.

Sip this tea during moonlit meditations to enhance your spiritual connection.

Words of Wisdom: "Like the moonlight, your inner light shines brightest in moments of stillness."

3. Empowerment Eucalyptus Bath Salts

Ingredients:

Epsom salt

Fresh eucalyptus leaves

A few drops of eucalyptus essential oil

Instructions:

Mix Epsom salt and fresh eucalyptus leaves in a bowl.

Add a few drops of eucalyptus essential oil.

Sprinkle these bath salts into your warm bath for empowerment and mental clarity.

Words of Wisdom: "Much like the eucalyptus, may your spirit soar with clarity and purpose."

4. Prosperity Potent Potpourri

Ingredients:

Dried cinnamon sticks

Dried bay leaves

Dried orange peel

Cloves

Instructions:

Combine dried cinnamon sticks, bay leaves, orange peel, and cloves.

Place this potent potpourri in a decorative dish in your sacred space.

Allow the aroma to fill the air, attracting prosperity and abundance.

Words of Wisdom: "Child, as the potpourri's fragrance fills your space, may prosperity fill your life."

5. Garden of Dreams Herbal Pillow

Ingredients:

Dried lavender flowers

Dried chamomile flowers

Small fabric pouch

Instructions:

Fill a small fabric pouch with dried lavender and chamomile flowers.

Place the herbal pillow under your regular pillow.

Enjoy restful and dream-filled nights.

Words of Wisdom: "Like the dreams nurtured in your pillow, may your aspirations take root and blossom."

6. Healing Herb-Infused Massage Oil

Ingredients:

Fresh calendula petals

Fresh comfrey leaves

Olive oil

Instructions:

Collect fresh calendula petals and comfrey leaves.

Place them in a glass jar and cover with olive oil.

Let it infuse in a sunny spot for 2-4 weeks.

Strain and use the herbal-infused oil for soothing massages.

Words of Wisdom: "Child, as this oil nurtures your body, nurture your spirit with self-love."

7. **Prosperity Protection Sachet**

Ingredients:

Dried rosemary

Dried basil

Dried thyme

Small fabric pouch

Instructions:

Combine dried rosemary, basil, and thyme.

Fill a small fabric pouch with the herbal mixture.

Carry this sachet with you for protection and to attract prosperity.

Words of Wisdom: "Just as the sachet shields, remember to protect your inner peace."

8. Herbal Harmony Meditation Incense

Ingredients:

Dried frankincense resin

Dried myrrh resin

Dried lavender

Dried rosemary

Instructions:

Mix dried frankincense, myrrh, lavender, and rosemary.

Burn this herbal incense during meditation to enhance inner harmony.

Words of Wisdom: "Like the rising incense, let your intentions ascend to the heavens."

9. Harmony Honey Elixir

Ingredients:

Fresh lemon balm leaves

Fresh thyme leaves

Raw honey

Instructions:

Harvest fresh lemon balm and thyme leaves.

Mix them with raw honey to create an elixir.

Take a spoonful daily to promote inner harmony and balance.

Words of Wisdom: "Child, like the harmony within this elixir, may your life be a symphony of peace."

10. **Words of Wisdom**

As my grandmother would lovingly remind me:

"Dear one, the healing garden is a reflection of the beauty within you. Just as you nurture these herbs and create sacred spaces, remember to nurture your inner sanctuary. Your intentions, like the plants, have the power to flourish and create harmony in your life. Trust in your own journey, and may your heart and spirit bloom."

With each herb you cultivate and each sacred space you create, may you find balance and harmony within yourself and your surroundings. Your inner garden is a place of infinite potential, so tend to it with love and intention.

Chapter 9: Herbal Wisdom for the Generations: Passing Down the Legacy

In my grandmother's garden, the legacy of herbal wisdom was a living testament to the enduring connection between generations. As I stood amidst the fragrant herbs and vibrant blossoms, I realized that this garden was not just a repository of knowledge; it was a sacred space where the wisdom of the past merged with the curiosity of the present, and where the art of herbalism was passed down from one generation to the next.

My grandmother had always emphasized the importance of sharing knowledge, of passing down the traditions and practices that had been cherished for centuries. Today, she said, was a day for me to carry that legacy forward—to become a steward of the herbal wisdom that had been lovingly imparted to me.

"Herbalism," my grandmother began, "is not just a solitary journey but a communal one. It is a tradition that has been carried through the ages, nurtured by the collective wisdom of our ancestors. Today, I shall share with you the importance of passing down this knowledge, for in doing so, we ensure that the art of herbalism continues to thrive."

With those words, my grandmother led me to a quiet corner of the garden, where a collection of journals and notebooks were carefully stacked on a wooden table. These were her journals—records of her herbal experiments, discoveries, and observations spanning decades.

The Wisdom of Journals

My grandmother explained that keeping a journal was an essential part of herbalism. "Journals," she said, "are our companions on the journey of herbal wisdom. They allow us to document our experiences, record our observations, and capture the subtle nuances of the plants."

As I leafed through her journals, I was struck by the meticulousness of her notes. Each entry was a treasure trove of information—details of plant growth, harvesting times, remedies crafted, and their effects on the body and soul.

"Journals," my grandmother continued, "are a bridge between generations. They ensure that the knowledge we gain is not lost but passed down to those who come after us. They are a testament to the ever-evolving journey of herbalism."

With her guidance, I began my own herbal journal—a blank canvas waiting to be filled with my experiences and insights. My grandmother encouraged me to document not only the remedies I crafted but also the stories and traditions that had been handed down through our family.

"Your journal," she said, "is a reflection of your unique path in herbalism. It is a record of your relationship with the plants, your discoveries, and your personal connection to this sacred art."

As I put pen to paper, I felt a sense of purpose—a commitment to carry forward the legacy of herbal wisdom that had been entrusted to me. My grandmother's journals had not only preserved her knowledge but had also provided a roadmap for my own journey.

The Healing Power of Storytelling

My grandmother often reminded me that herbalism was not just about the physical remedies but also about the stories and traditions that surrounded them. She believed that storytelling was a powerful way to convey knowledge, to create connections, and to pass down the wisdom of the plants.

"Stories," she said, "have a way of touching the heart and soul. They make knowledge relatable and memorable. Today, I shall share with you some of the stories that have been woven into our family's herbal traditions."

She began with a tale of the healing properties of rosemary—a herb renowned for its ability to enhance memory and cognition. In ancient Greece, she explained, students would wear wreaths of rosemary while studying for exams, believing that it would help them retain knowledge. This story illustrated the deep connection between folklore and the therapeutic properties of plants.

Next, my grandmother recounted a family story about the calming effects of chamomile. She described how, during times of stress or restlessness, her own grandmother would brew a pot of chamomile tea and gather the family around. As they sipped the tea and shared stories, a sense of calm and unity would settle over them. This narrative highlighted the emotional and communal aspects of herbal remedies.

"Stories," my grandmother said, "are a way to pass down not only knowledge but also the essence of herbalism—the deep connection between humans and the natural world, the healing power of intention, and the importance of community and sharing."

With her encouragement, I began to collect and document the stories that had been part of our family's herbal traditions. These stories were not just anecdotes but vessels of wisdom that carried the heart and soul of herbalism.

The Role of Mentorship

One of the most profound aspects of herbalism, my grandmother explained, was the relationship between mentor and student. She believed that mentorship was a vital part of passing down the legacy of herbal wisdom.

"As a mentor," she said, "I have had the privilege of guiding you on this journey, just as I was guided by my own mentors. Mentorship is a sacred exchange of knowledge, trust, and wisdom."

My grandmother shared stories of her own mentors—herbalists and wise women who had imparted their knowledge and traditions to her. She described how these mentors had not only taught her about plants but had also instilled in her a deep respect for the earth, a sense of wonder for the natural world, and an understanding of the interconnectedness of all living beings.

"As you continue on your path," she said, "I encourage you to seek out mentors who can offer guidance, wisdom, and a deeper understanding of herbalism. Mentorship is a journey of growth and transformation, and it ensures that the legacy of herbalism remains vibrant and alive."

With her words in mind, I began to actively seek out herbalists and practitioners who could serve as mentors. Each mentor brought a unique perspective, a wealth of experience, and a deep connection to the plants. They not only expanded my knowledge but also enriched my understanding of the diverse traditions within herbalism.

Teaching the Next Generation

As our day in the garden drew to a close, my grandmother turned her gaze toward the future. "Passing down the legacy of herbal wisdom," she said, "is not just about preserving the past but also about nurturing the generations to come. It is our responsibility to ensure that this knowledge continues to thrive."

She explained that teaching the next generation was a vital part of this legacy. "Just as I have shared this journey with you," she said, "you, too, will have the opportunity to teach and inspire others. Through teaching, we reinforce our own knowledge and become a link in the chain of wisdom."

With her guidance, I began to share my knowledge with younger family members and friends who expressed an interest in herbalism. We gathered in the garden, and I shared stories, remedies, and traditions, just as my grandmother had done with me.

"Teaching," my grandmother said, "is a way to give back to the community and to ensure that the legacy of herbalism continues to flourish. It is a way to honor the wisdom of our ancestors and to celebrate the beauty, wonder, and interconnectedness of the natural world."

In the heart of the garden, I had not only learned the art of herbalism but also the importance of passing down the legacy of wisdom, knowledge, and tradition. It was a journey that extended beyond the confines of the garden and into the very heart of nature itself—a journey that celebrated the enduring magic of herbalism, the interconnectedness of all living beings, and the deep reverence for the wisdom of the plants.

1. **Generational Healing Tincture**

Ingredients:

Fresh elderberries

Fresh echinacea leaves and flowers

Brandy or vodka

Instructions:

Gather fresh elderberries and echinacea leaves and flowers.

Place them in a glass jar and cover with brandy or vodka.

Let it steep for at least six weeks.

Share this tincture with your family to boost immunity and pass down the healing tradition.

Words of Wisdom: "Child, as we share this tincture, remember that healing is a gift meant to be passed from one generation to the next."

2. Ancestral Herbal Storytelling Tea

Ingredients:

1 tablespoon dried hawthorn berries

1 tablespoon dried nettle leaves

1 teaspoon dried mugwort

A pinch of dried lemon balm

Boiling water

Instructions:

In a teapot, blend hawthorn berries, nettle leaves, mugwort, and lemon balm.

Pour boiling water over the herbs and let steep for 10-15 minutes.

Share this tea with your loved ones while sharing stories of herbal wisdom from your family's past.

Words of Wisdom: "Child, as we sip this tea and share stories, remember that our heritage is a tapestry woven with love and knowledge."

3. **Herbal Legacy Healing Balm**

Ingredients:

Fresh comfrey leaves

Fresh calendula petals

Beeswax

Olive oil

Instructions:

Collect fresh comfrey leaves and calendula petals.

Melt beeswax in a double boiler.

Add comfrey leaves and calendula petals to create a healing balm.

Share this balm with your family to pass on the tradition of natural healing.

Words of Wisdom: "Much like the healing balm, our family's legacy is a salve for the soul."

4. Generations of Love Infused Honey

Ingredients:

Fresh rose petals

Raw honey

Instructions:

Harvest fresh rose petals from your garden.

Mix the petals with raw honey to create an infused honey.

Allow it to sit for a few weeks.

Share this honey with your family to pass down the tradition of love and care.

Words of Wisdom: "Child, like the sweet embrace of honey, let love be the foundation of our family."

5. Herbal Mentorship Elixir

Ingredients:

Fresh lemon balm leaves

Fresh thyme leaves

Raw honey

Instructions:

Harvest fresh lemon balm and thyme leaves.

Mix them with raw honey to create an elixir.

Share this elixir with a younger family member, passing on the knowledge and wisdom of herbalism.

Words of Wisdom: "Just as I mentored you, pass on the torch of knowledge to the next generation."

6. **Wisdom Journal Herbal Tea**

Ingredients:

1 tablespoon dried sage leaves

1 tablespoon dried rosemary leaves

1 teaspoon dried lemon balm

A pinch of dried lavender

Boiling water

Instructions:

In a teapot, blend sage leaves, rosemary leaves, lemon balm, and lavender.

Pour boiling water over the herbs and let steep for 10-15 minutes.

Sip this tea while journaling about your herbal experiences and knowledge to create a wisdom journal to share with future generations.

Words of Wisdom: "Child, as you write in your journal, remember that knowledge is a torch that lights the path for others."

7. Herbal Wisdom Bath Salts

Ingredients:

Epsom salt

Dried chamomile flowers

Dried rose petals

A few drops of lavender essential oil

Instructions:

Mix Epsom salt, dried chamomile flowers, and dried rose petals in a bowl.

Add a few drops of lavender essential oil.

Share these bath salts with a younger family member, encouraging them to connect with nature's healing power.

Words of Wisdom: "Like the bath salts, our heritage is a blend of soothing wisdom and fragrant stories."

8. Tea of Generations

Ingredients:

1 tablespoon dried elderberries

1 tablespoon dried hibiscus petals

1 teaspoon dried nettle leaves

A pinch of dried mint

Boiling water

Instructions:

In a teapot, combine elderberries, hibiscus petals, nettle leaves, and mint.

Pour boiling water over the herbs and let steep for 10-15 minutes.

Share this tea with your family, passing on the tradition of herbal remedies.

Words of Wisdom: "Child, as we sip this tea, let it be a reminder of our family's strong roots and nurturing love."

9. **Healing Garden Meditation Incense**

Ingredients:

Dried lavender

Dried rosemary

Dried sage

Dried thyme

Instructions:

Mix dried lavender, rosemary, sage, and thyme.

Burn this herbal incense during family meditations to connect with nature's healing energies.

Words of Wisdom: "Like the rising incense, let our family's spirit ascend with each generation."

10. **Words of Wisdom**

As my grandmother would lovingly remind me:

"Dear one, the herbal wisdom we hold is a treasure meant to be shared. Just as we have nurtured the healing traditions, you too must be a keeper of the flame. Pass on the knowledge, love, and stories to those who follow, and may our family's legacy be a beacon of light in their lives."

With each shared remedy and story, you preserve our family's heritage and empower the generations to come. The wisdom you carry is a gift, and it is your responsibility to pass it on, so that the herbal flame continues to burn brightly.

Chapter 10: The Healing Garden: Cultivating Herbal Harmony

In my grandmother's garden, the true essence of herbalism lay not only in the individual remedies and knowledge but also in the art of cultivating a healing garden—a space where plants, people, and the natural world harmoniously coexisted. It was a sanctuary of greenery, a tapestry of colors and fragrances, and a living testament to the power of nature's remedies.

My grandmother had always emphasized that herbalism was not just a practice but a way of life—a deep reverence for the earth and an understanding of our role as stewards of the land. As I walked through the garden, I realized that this sacred space was not just a collection of plants; it was a living entity—a partner in the journey of healing and well-being.

"Today," my grandmother said, her eyes twinkling with excitement, "we shall explore the art of creating a healing garden—a place where the wisdom of the plants comes to life, where we cultivate harmony with nature, and where we can connect with the healing energies of the earth."

With those words, she led me to a quiet corner of the garden, where a lush, vibrant patch of herbs and flowers thrived. This, she explained, was her healing garden—a place where she cultivated the plants that held special significance for her and our family.

The Healing Garden: A Sanctuary of Intentions

My grandmother began our lesson by explaining the concept of a healing garden.

"A healing garden," she said, "is more than just a collection of herbs. It is a space where intention meets nature—a sanctuary where the plants are not just cultivated but cherished, where their healing energies are harnessed, and where we can commune with the earth."

She emphasized the importance of intention in creating a healing garden. "Before we even plant a single seed," she said, "we must set our intentions for the garden. What is the purpose of this space? Is it for physical healing, emotional solace, or spiritual connection? Our intentions shape the energy of the garden."

With her guidance, we sat in the garden and closed our eyes. My grandmother encouraged me to connect with the energy of the earth, to visualize the garden as a place of healing and transformation, and to set my own intentions for the space.

"As you cultivate your healing garden," she said, "remember that it is a reflection of your own journey—a mirror of your connection to the earth and your commitment to holistic well-being."

As we opened our eyes, I felt a profound sense of connection to the garden—an understanding that it was not just a physical space but a living entity that responded to our intentions and care.

Planting with Purpose: Choosing the Right Herbs

The heart of a healing garden, my grandmother explained, lay in the selection of plants. "Choosing the right herbs," she said, "is like composing a symphony. Each plant brings its unique qualities to the garden, contributing to the overall harmony and healing potential."

We started with herbs that had special significance to our family. Lemon balm, for instance, was a beloved herb that had been used for generations to soothe frayed nerves and promote a sense of calm. We planted it near a quiet bench, where its fragrance could be enjoyed during moments of reflection.

Calendula, with its vibrant orange blossoms, was another family favorite known for its skin-healing properties. We planted it near the garden's entrance, a reminder of the healing potential that awaited those who entered.

"Planting with purpose," my grandmother said, "is about aligning the qualities of the herbs with the intentions of the garden. It is a deliberate act of co-creation with nature."

We selected herbs that represented various aspects of healing—lavender for emotional well-being, echinacea for immune support, and chamomile for inner peace. Each herb found its place in the garden, contributing to the overall tapestry of healing energies.

Designing a Healing Space

The layout of a healing garden was not just a matter of aesthetics but an essential aspect of its functionality. My grandmother explained that the design of the garden should promote a sense of balance and harmony.

Paths were carefully laid out to allow easy access to all parts of the garden, ensuring that no plant was neglected. The garden was divided into themed sections—areas for relaxation, meditation, and herb gathering. Each section served a specific purpose, creating a multifaceted space for healing and connection.

"A healing garden," my grandmother said, "should be a place of serenity and tranquility. It should invite people to slow down, connect with the plants, and find solace in the embrace of nature."

We added benches and stone seating areas, where visitors could sit and meditate, journal, or simply immerse themselves in the beauty of the garden. Wind chimes and bird feeders were strategically placed to attract wildlife, adding to the sense of natural harmony.

"Designing a healing space," my grandmother emphasized, "is about creating an environment that nurtures the body, mind, and spirit. It should be a haven where people can find respite from the demands of daily life and tap into the healing energies of the earth."

Caring for the Garden: A Partnership with Nature

Cultivating a healing garden, my grandmother explained, was an ongoing partnership with nature. It required not only planting and design but also mindful care and stewardship.

"Taking care of the garden," she said, "is a daily practice of presence and mindfulness. It is about tuning into the rhythms of nature, observing the needs of the plants, and nurturing the soil and ecosystem."

We tended to the garden with care, watering the plants, weeding, and ensuring that each herb received the attention it deserved. My grandmother emphasized the importance of organic and sustainable practices, using natural fertilizers and compost to nourish the soil.

"By caring for the garden," she said, "we are also caring for ourselves. The act of tending to the plants, of connecting with the earth, is a form of meditation and self-care."

As I worked in the garden, I felt a deep sense of connection to the earth—a recognition that I was not just a caretaker but a part of the garden's ecosystem. The garden responded to our care with vibrant growth, fragrant blossoms, and a sense of vitality that permeated the space.

Harvesting and Using the Garden's Bounty

One of the most rewarding aspects of a healing garden was the opportunity to harvest and use its bounty. My grandmother showed me how to harvest herbs at their peak, ensuring that their healing properties were preserved.

"Harvesting," she explained, "is a sacred act of gratitude. It is a recognition of the gifts that the plants offer us and a way to honor their energy and wisdom."

We harvested herbs for teas, tinctures, and salves, always taking care to leave some plants to continue growing and thriving. My grandmother emphasized the importance of sustainable harvesting, ensuring that the garden remained abundant for generations to come.

"Using the garden's bounty," she said, "is a way to bring its healing energies into our lives. It is a direct connection to the earth and a reminder of the power of nature's remedies."

As we prepared remedies from the garden's herbs, I felt a profound sense of connection to the plants and to the wisdom they held. It was a reminder that the healing journey extended beyond the garden's boundaries and into the very essence of our daily lives.

Sharing the Healing Garden

My grandmother had always believed that the healing garden was not just for personal use but a gift to be shared with others. She encouraged me to open the garden to family, friends, and the community, inviting them to experience its healing energies.

"Sharing the healing garden," she said, "is a way to spread the wisdom of herbalism, to connect with others on their healing journeys, and to create a sense of community and belonging."

We hosted gatherings in the garden—herbal workshops, meditation sessions, and tea ceremonies. Visitors would walk through the garden's paths, touching the leaves, inhaling the fragrances, and connecting with the plants in a profound way.

"Through the healing garden," my grandmother said, "we offer a space of solace, inspiration, and transformation. It is a way to give back to the earth and to the people who seek healing and connection."

As I watched the garden become a place of shared wisdom and communal healing, I realized that it was not just a sanctuary for me and my grandmother but a gift to the world—a reminder of the healing potential that lay within the embrace of nature.

The Healing Garden as a Legacy

As our day in the garden came to a close, my grandmother turned to me with a smile. "The healing garden," she said, "is a legacy—a testament to our love for the earth, our commitment to well-being, and our connection to the wisdom of the plants. It is a living entity that will continue to thrive long after we are gone."

She explained that a healing garden was not just a physical space but a reflection of our values and intentions—a testament to our belief in the healing power of nature and our dedication to passing down this wisdom to future generations.

"In the heart of the healing garden," my grandmother said, "we find the essence of herbalism—a journey that extends beyond the confines of the garden and into the very heart of nature itself. It is a journey of cultivation, intention, and a deep reverence for the enduring magic of herbalism—a world where healing is not just a matter of science and medicine but a sacred art that celebrates the beauty, wonder, and interconnectedness of the natural world."

As I stood in the garden, I knew that it was a legacy I would carry with me throughout my life—a reminder of the healing potential that lay within the embrace of nature, a commitment to stewardship of the earth, and a deep reverence for the wisdom of the plants. It was a legacy that would continue to flourish, nurturing the body, mind, and spirit, and serving as a testament to the enduring magic of the healing garden.

1. **Eternal Garden Tea**

Ingredients:

1 tablespoon dried rose petals

1 tablespoon dried lemon balm leaves

1 teaspoon dried chamomile flowers

A pinch of dried lavender

Boiling water

Instructions:

In a teapot, blend rose petals, lemon balm leaves, chamomile flowers, and lavender.

Pour boiling water over the herbs and let steep for 10-15 minutes.

Sip this tea while contemplating the everlasting connection between the garden and your legacy.

Words of Wisdom: "Child, as you enjoy this tea, remember that our love for the garden will live on through you."

2. **Family Herbal Potent Potion**

Ingredients:

Fresh comfrey leaves

Fresh mint leaves

Raw honey

Brandy or vodka

Instructions:

Harvest fresh comfrey leaves and mint leaves.

Place them in a glass jar and cover with brandy or vodka.

Let it steep for at least six weeks.

Add raw honey to taste and share this potent potion with family, ensuring that our herbal legacy thrives.

Words of Wisdom: "Much like this potion, the love for healing herbs flows through our veins."

3. **Generations of Well-Being Salve**

Ingredients:

Fresh calendula flowers

Fresh plantain leaves

Beeswax

Olive oil

Instructions:

Collect fresh calendula flowers and plantain leaves.

Melt beeswax in a double boiler.

Add the herbs to create a soothing salve.

Pass this salve down to the next generation, nurturing their well-being and connection to the earth.

Words of Wisdom: "Child, as you use this salve, remember that our herbal legacy heals not only the body but also the spirit."

4. Prosperity Protection Amulet

Ingredients:

Small fabric pouch

Dried rosemary

Dried bay leaves

Small citrine crystal

Instructions:

Fill a small fabric pouch with dried rosemary, bay leaves, and a small citrine crystal.

Carry this amulet with you to protect your legacy and invite prosperity.

Words of Wisdom: "Just as the amulet guards, protect the garden of your soul."

5. Herbal Harmony Anointing Oil

Ingredients:

Fresh rose petals

Fresh lavender flowers

Olive oil

Instructions:

Harvest fresh rose petals and lavender flowers.

Place them in a glass jar and cover with olive oil.

Let it infuse in sunlight for 2-4 weeks.

Share this anointing oil with loved ones, passing down the legacy of herbal harmony.

Words of Wisdom: "Much like the oil's fragrance, may our herbal legacy permeate every aspect of life."

6. Legacy-Enriching Herbal Elixir

Ingredients:

Fresh St. John's Wort flowers

Fresh meadowsweet leaves and flowers

Raw honey

Instructions:

Harvest fresh St. John's Wort flowers and meadowsweet leaves and flowers.

Mix them with raw honey to create an elixir.

Share this elixir with family members, nurturing the legacy of well-being.

Words of Wisdom: "Child, as you sip this elixir, remember that our legacy is woven with threads of health and happiness."

7. Wisdom Garden Meditation Incense

Ingredients:

Dried sage

Dried rosemary

Dried lavender

Dried thyme

Instructions:

Mix dried sage, rosemary, lavender, and thyme.

Burn this herbal incense during family meditations, connecting with the wisdom passed down through generations.

Words of Wisdom: "Like the rising incense, let the wisdom of our garden rise in your heart."

8. Legacy of Love Herbal Sachet

Ingredients:

Dried lavender buds

Dried rose petals

Small fabric pouch

Instructions:

Combine dried lavender buds and rose petals.

Fill a small fabric pouch with the herbal mixture.

Place it in your home to keep the legacy of love alive.

Words of Wisdom: "Child, as you hold this sachet, remember that love is our most cherished legacy."

9. Garden of Wisdom Botanical Book

Ingredients:

Blank journal

Pressed flowers and herbs

Family herbal wisdom

Instructions:

Create a botanical book by pressing flowers and herbs between its pages.

Share your family's herbal wisdom and stories in this book.

Pass it on to the next generation, ensuring the garden's wisdom lives on.

Words of Wisdom: "Much like the pages of this book, our family's knowledge is an enduring legacy."

10. **Words of Wisdom**

As my grandmother would lovingly remind me:

"Dear one, the healing garden is a legacy that transcends time. As you nurture its growth, remember that the love and knowledge we've shared will flourish in your care. Continue to honor the earth and the healing gifts it offers. Our herbal legacy is a testament to our connection to nature and our commitment to the well-being of generations to come."

With each plant you tend and each remedy you create, you carry forth the heritage of our family's herbal wisdom. The garden is a living legacy, and you are its keeper.

Dear cherished readers,

As I reflect on the journey we've embarked on together through the pages of "My Grandmother's Witchy Medicine Cabinet," I am filled with profound gratitude for each of you who have embraced this magical odyssey of herbalism and healing. Your support and curiosity have breathed life into the ancient wisdom passed down through generations, and for that, I am truly thankful.

I hope that the knowledge shared within these chapters has opened new doorways of understanding and reverence for the natural world around us. The art and magic of herbalism are not confined to the past; they are living, breathing practices that can illuminate our path toward well-being in the present and the future.

As we part ways for now, I offer you these words of wisdom: Embrace the future with a heart filled with hope and the wisdom that every day is an opportunity to grow, heal, and connect with the beauty of the world around you. Just as the seasons change, so do our lives, and within that change, there is a constant wellspring of possibility.

May you continue to explore the healing energies
of herbs, to tend your own sacred apothecary, and
to nurture the deep connection between yourself
and the natural world. You hold the power to heal,
to transform, and to create a legacy of well-being
for generations to come.

Thank you for being a part of this journey, and may
your path be filled with blessings, love, and the
boundless magic of herbalism.

With heartfelt gratitude,

A.L. Childers

Appendices: Your Herbal Companion

In our journey through "My Grandmother's Witchy Medicine Cabinet," we have explored the enchanting world of herbalism—a realm where nature's remedies and ancestral wisdom converge to promote holistic well-being. This appendices section serves as your herbal companion, offering an array of resources, recommendations, recipes, and a glossary to enhance your understanding and exploration of herbalism.

Appendix A: Resources for Further Learning

Embarking on a journey of herbal wisdom is a lifelong pursuit. This section provides you with an extensive list of resources to further your education and deepen your connection to herbalism. Whether you're seeking books, websites, courses, or organizations, these resources are your compass in navigating the vast landscape of herbal knowledge.

Books for Herbal Education

"The Herbal Medicine-Maker's Handbook" by James Green

"Rosemary Gladstar's Medicinal Herbs: A Beginner's Guide" by Rosemary Gladstar

"The Modern Herbal Dispensatory: A Medicine-Making Guide" by Thomas Easley and Steven Horne

"The Complete Illustrated Holistic Herbal: A Safe and Practical Guide to Making and Using Herbal Remedies" by David Hoffmann

"The Earthwise Herbal: A Complete Guide to Old World Medicinal Plants" by Matthew Wood

Websites for Herbal Reference

Herbal Academy

American Herbalists Guild

United Plant Savers

Mountain Rose Herbs Blog

The Herbalist's Path

Online Courses

The Herbal Academy

The Chestnut School of Herbal Medicine

East West School of Planetary Herbology

Northwest School for Botanical Studies

The School of Evolutionary Herbalism

Herbal Organizations

American Herbalists Guild

United Plant Savers

International Herb Association

American Botanical Council

Herb Society of America

Appendix B: Additional Reading Recommendations and Educational Resources

Explore a curated selection of additional reading recommendations and educational resources to deepen your understanding of herbalism and its diverse facets. These texts and materials offer insights into specialized topics and perspectives that complement the journey you've embarked upon.

Additional Reading Recommendations

"The Lost Language of Plants: The Ecological Importance of Plant Medicines to Life on Earth" by Stephen Harrod Buhner

"The Secret Teachings of Plants: The Intelligence of the Heart in the Direct Perception of Nature" by Stephen Harrod Buhner

"Plant Spirit Medicine: A Journey into the Healing Wisdom of Plants" by Eliot Cowan

"The Wild Medicine Solution: Healing with Aromatic, Bitter, and Tonic Plants" by Guido Masé

"Alchemy of Herbs: Transform Everyday Ingredients into Foods and Remedies That Heal" by Rosalee de la Forêt

Educational Resources

YouTube Channel: Herbal Jedi

Herbal Radio Podcast

The Plant Path Podcast

HerbMentor

Herbal Roots Zine

Appendix C: Recipes for Herbal Remedies and Potions

Dive into the world of herbal alchemy with a collection of detailed, step-by-step recipes for creating the herbal remedies and potions discussed in the book. These recipes are infused with personal anecdotes and insights from my own experiences in making and using these remedies.

Calming Chamomile Tea

A soothing infusion to calm nerves and promote relaxation.

Elderberry Syrup

A potent immune-boosting elixir to ward off colds and flu.

Comfrey Salve

A healing balm for skin irritations and minor wounds.

Lavender and Rosemary Hair Rinse

A fragrant blend to promote healthy hair and a calm mind.

Echinacea Tincture

An immune-enhancing potion for warding off infections.

Minty Digestive Bitters

A digestive aid to alleviate indigestion and promote healthy digestion.

Rose Petal Elixir

A heart-opening elixir to soothe the emotions and nurture self-love.

Sage and Thyme Respiratory Steam

A comforting steam for congestion and respiratory relief.

Appendix D: Glossary of Herbal Terms

Navigating the language of herbalism can be akin to deciphering a mystical script. This glossary provides definitions and explanations of key herbal terminology, ensuring that you have a handy reference for understanding the intricate world of herbs.

Common Herbal Terms

Infusion: A method of extracting the therapeutic properties of herbs by steeping them in hot water.

Tincture: A concentrated herbal extract made by soaking herbs in alcohol or glycerin.

Decoction: A method of extracting herbal properties by boiling the herbs in water.

Infusion vs. Decoction: Understanding the difference between these two methods of extraction.

Adaptogen: A substance that helps the body adapt to stress and maintain balance.

Aromatic: Herbs that have a strong fragrance and often contain volatile oils.

Demulcent: Herbs that soothe and protect mucous membranes.

Emollient: Herbs or substances that soften and soothe the skin.

Antispasmodic: Herbs that relieve muscle spasms and cramps.

Alterative: Herbs that gradually restore health and vitality to the body.

Pronunciations and Etymology

Echinacea: Pronounced eh-kih-NAY-see-uh, derived from the Greek word "echinos," meaning hedgehog, due to the spiky center of the flower.

Comfrey: Pronounced KUM-free, derived from the Latin "confera," meaning "to bring together" due to its traditional use in healing wounds.

Calendula: Pronounced kuh-LEN-dyoo-luh, derived from the Latin "calendae," meaning "first day of the month," due to its prolific flowering.

Rosmarinus officinalis: Pronounced rohs-muh-REE-nuhs oh-fuh-SIN-uh-lis, derived from Latin, meaning "dew of the sea," alluding to its habitat.

Hypericum perforatum: Pronounced hi-PER-ih-kum per-for-AY-tum, derived from Greek, meaning "over an apparition" due to its traditional use in warding off evil spirits.

With these appendices, you hold a treasure trove of knowledge and practical guidance to embark on your own herbal journey. Whether you are a novice or seasoned herbalist, may this resource enhance your exploration of the healing world of plants, connecting you to the timeless wisdom of "My Grandmother's Witchy Medicine Cabinet." As you continue to unlock the secrets of herbalism, may the vibrant tapestry of nature's remedies enrich your life and foster a deeper connection to the earth and its abundant gifts.